S0-ACU-096

THE SECRET LANGUAGE OF DOCTORS

The Secret Language
of Doctors

CRACKING THE CODE OF HOSPITAL CULTURE

////////////////////////////

DR. BRIAN GOLDMAN

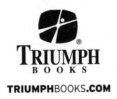

TRIUMPHBOOKS.COM

The Secret Language of Doctors
Copyright © 2014 by Brian Goldman Enterprises Ltd.
All rights reserved.

No part of this book may be reproduced, stored in a retrieval system, or transmitted
in any form by any means, electronic, mechanical, photocopying, or otherwise,
without the prior written permission of the publisher, Triumph Books LLC,
814 North Franklin Street, Chicago, Illinois 60610.

This book is available in quantity at special dicounts for your group or organization.

For further information, contact:
Triumph Books LLC
814 North Franklin Street
Chicago, Illinois 60610
Phone: (312) 337-0747
www.triumphbooks.com

Printed in the United States of America

ISBN 978-1-62937-092-7

Published simultaneously in Canada by HarperCollins Publishers Ltd.

To my late father, Samuel, who died before he could read this book, and to my mother, Shirley, whose heart is in this book though she'll never read it.

Contents

THE SECRET LANGUAGE OF DOCTORS

The Bunker

6 *p.m. Handover*
In a small, secluded room behind the nursing station of Ward 6 West, residents gather for the daily ritual called handover, or patient sign-out. It's the moment when the army of staff doing scheduled tests, interventions and operations shifts down to a skeleton crew of residents on call whose job is to monitor patients and attend to any sudden emergencies. It's also when residents who aren't on call finally get to go home. But first, they have to give their colleagues the heads-up on every patient under their charge.

The rectangular room where they meet is nicknamed the Bunker. The room contains four cubicles equipped with computers, a printer and a coffee machine. A small sofa bed is off to one side. The walls' blue paint is scuffed with furniture marks. In the middle of the room is a small conference table ringed with chairs.

The Bunker is where residents meet with the ward chief—the attending or most senior physician in charge of the patients—to write up chart notes and to talk frankly about patients and fellow doctors who work on other floors and in other hospitals. The room, teeming with two sets of residents—the ones on call and the ones handing over—is hot and stuffy.

"Room 22, bed B, 82-year-old male," says Rick, a first-year resident in internal medicine. "Admitted ten days ago with a fractured pelvis. He also has moderate Alzheimer's dementia, GERD and type 2 diabetes. OT and PT say it's not safe for him to go home. He's awaiting placement."

"What's his code status?" asks Sandi, the senior resident on call.

"He's Full Code," answers Rick. "We tried to get the DNR but the family said they're thinking about it."

"Thinking about it?" repeats Sandi. "Can we do a Hollywood Code?"

"You're on call, so it's your show," says Raza, the senior resident on Rick's team. "But the family is there 24/7. I think they'd know it if you run a Slow Code."

"You may hear about a consult we did on ortho," says Raza. "Eighty-eight-year-old female five days post right total hip replacement. Post-op, she was overhydrated by the ortho resident and put into CHF. She had a bump in her troponin. We've given her Lasix and she's feeling better. She's stable now."

"Saved another FOOBA," says Sandi.

"That's the third one this month," says Raza.

"Next patient is Room 24, bed C, 58-year-old female," says Rick. "Admitted over the weekend with type 1 diabetes and DKA triggered by a urinary tract infection. Unfortunately, she developed a pressure sore on her sacrum. Plastics is consulting on that."

"Pressure ulcer?" asks Sandi. "How the hell does a 58-year-old diabetic get a pressure ulcer on her bum?"

"She's a beemer," says Raza.

"How big is she?" asks Sandi.

"Three clinic units," answers Raza. "We tried using the Hoyer lift but it wasn't rated for her."

"Sounds like a horrendoma," says Sandi.

"It gets worse," says Rick. "We don't have a bariatric commode or wheelchair to get her to the bathroom. She had a Code Brown in the bed."

"Who got to clean that up?" asks Sandi.

"Thank god for LPNs," says Raza. Everybody in the room laughs.

////////

The dialogue you just read was created to illustrate just how much medical jargon can be packed into a brief discussion.

The 82-year-old man has GERD, which stands for gastroesophageal reflux disease, better known as heartburn. The residents referred him to OT and PT—occupational therapy and physiotherapy. That's standard procedure for a patient with a cracked pelvis to determine whether the fracture will keep him from going home; an OT/PT assessment is also used to find out if a patient is likely to fall at home and what preventative safety measures might be necessary.

Raza's 88-year-old patient on the orthopedic floor went into CHF—congestive heart failure—after the orthopedic resident gave her too much intravenous fluid. A "bump in her troponin" means the woman had a slight increase in the level of a protein called troponin, which indicates that she suffered a mild heart attack.

The 58-year-old woman was admitted to hospital with DKA, which stands for diabetic ketoacidosis, a life-threatening condition in which both the sugar and acid in the bloodstream rise to dangerous levels. A "plastics consult" means she was seen by a plastic surgeon, the specialist who usually manages skin ulcers.

But the residents also used a bunch of words and phrases that aren't found in any medical textbook I know of, yet they were understood by everyone in the Bunker. If you sat in on that conversation, you might have thought you'd wandered into a very boring French film. Now, let's provide the subtitles—starting with the 82-year-old man.

- "He's awaiting placement" means there are no ongoing medical issues and if he could go home safely, we'd have sent him out by now.
- "What's his code status?" means "Do we have to do CPR (cardiopulmonary resuscitation) if his heart stops?"
- "He's Full Code. We tried to get the DNR but the family said they're thinking about it" means the family wants him to be resuscitated if his heart stops. They can't see the handwriting on the wall—that there's no point in doing CPR if his heart stops—and they aren't ready to sign a Do Not Resuscitate order.
- "Can we do a Hollywood Code?" means that if his heart stops we'll do a pretend resuscitation in which it looks as if we're trying to save him but we aren't.

Now, we'll take look at the acronym Sandi the resident used to talk about the patient on the orthopedic floor who was put into congestive heart failure. "Saved another FOOBA" means the internal medicine team saved another patient who was "found on orthopedics barely alive." It's a dig at orthopedic surgeons, who have a reputation for being so focused on what needs to be fixed surgically that they ignore signs of other diseases. FOOBA is a play on FUBAR, a military slang term that has entered common vernacular and stands for "fucked up beyond all repair."

Finally, let's unpack the slang that was used by the residents to talk about the 58-year-old woman in Room 24, bed C:

- "How the hell does a 58-year-old diabetic get a pressure ulcer on her bum?—She's a beemer" means the woman got a pressure ulcer on her buttocks because she has a high body mass index, or BMI, a polite way of saying that she is morbidly obese. In other words, she's so large that she developed a pressure ulcer from lying on her backside too long because she was too weak to move and she weighed too much for nurses to shift her position in bed.
- "Three clinic units" is a sneaky way of saying the patient weighs 600 pounds. One clinic unit refers to a weight of 200 pounds.
- "Sounds like a horrendoma" refers to a horrible or awful condition.
- "We don't have a bariatric commode or wheelchair to get her to the bathroom. She had a Code Brown in the bed" means that she is so large that when she had to defecate, several nurses—who didn't have special lifting equipment—could not manage to move her to the bathroom or commode or even to place a bedpan underneath her, so she defecated in her bed.
- "Thank god for LPNs" refers to licensed practical nurses. Poop runs downhill. Residents can laugh about a Code Brown because they aren't the ones who have to clean it up.

That is a crash course in the Secret Language of Doctors and what the language reveals about how these doctors view patients and their families in the culture of modern medicine.

//////

Doctors share a culture that many hardly realize exists, much less talk about. In a 2008 paper published in the journal *Academic Medicine*,

Dr. Carla Boutin-Foster and colleagues defined medical culture as "the language, thought processes, styles of communication, customs, and beliefs that often characterize the profession of medicine."

Much of what is written about the culture of medicine focuses on the qualities of the ideal physician—what Boutin-Foster listed as "honesty, empathy, altruism, honor, and respect." These attributes are considered the core values of medical professionalism. The doctor's white coat is a powerful symbol of medical culture. Many medical schools hold a White Coat Ceremony during which first year students receive a white coat along with a lecture that teaches positive cultural values to young doctors to be.

But, there's another side to medical culture—one that reflects how doctors cope with the not-so-nice aspects of medicine—everything from exhaustion and sleep deprivation to frustrations with Obamacare, not to mention frustration with certain kinds of patients and families, fellow doctors and allied health professionals.

They share these feelings only with trusted colleagues. To know what they really think about you, a loved one, or the heart surgeon about to remove a cancer inside your belly, you'd have to eavesdrop on conversations that take place away from the bedside.

///////

To understand what you're hearing, it helps to learn a little bit of "medical slang." A more accurate term is *argot* (pronounced "argo"), which is defined by the *Merriam-Webster Dictionary* as "an often more or less secret vocabulary and idiom peculiar to a particular group." The purpose of argot is to prevent eavesdropping outsiders from understanding what you're talking about and to create a bond among colleagues, teammates or friends.

Argot is a French word. According to linguist Pierre Guiraud, the first known record of the word is in a document written in 1628; Guiraud wrote that *argot* was derived from *les argotiers*, a name then given to a group of thieves. In his 1862 novel *Les Misérables*, Victor Hugo described argot as "the language of misery." As you will discover in this book, that description fits with the experience of residents and sometimes of other medical staff working in hospitals.

Argot is also sometimes referred to as a cant or cryptolect. The Thieves' Cant—a secret language used by robbers and other criminals—was popularized in theatre and pamphlets during the late sixteenth and early seventeenth centuries. Today *argot* is used to describe the informal and highly specialized nomenclature and vocabulary used by people in a particular occupation, hobby, sport or field of study.

An argot comes not just with a unique vocabulary but also with its own grammar and syntax. If you were to overhear two physicians speaking medical argot in an elevator, you might have trouble understanding what they were saying. But you'd probably be able to recognize that they were speaking English. Medical argot is simply English augmented with code words that are incomprehensible to all but initiates.

⁄⁄⁄⁄⁄⁄⁄

My introduction to the secret language of doctors came when I was fresh out of medical school in 1980 and doing a year of residency in pediatrics at the Hospital for Sick Children in Toronto. Residents are new graduates of medical schools taking postgraduate training in everything from family medicine to neurosurgery. At one point, I had chosen a career treating children with disorders of the brain and had to do at least three years of training in general pediatrics before embarking on the "final" stage of my career development. However, within six months I abandoned that career choice entirely, in no small part because of the suffering I experienced as a young resident.

On average, I worked seventy to eighty hours a week, from 8 a.m. until 6 p.m. on weekdays, plus one night in three on call. If I was on call for the weekend, it was more like 110 hours for the week. Being on call meant that I stayed overnight in the hospital while my fellow residents went home. That meant I was responsible overnight for my patients and for theirs. In addition, anywhere from four to ten times a night I had to go down to the emergency department to admit patients assigned to my ward.

The nights on call were gruelling and relentless. I can remember running from one sick baby or child to the next, with little time even for a pee break. In addition to the volume of work, when you're treating very ill babies and children there's often a greater sense of anxiety than there is when you are treating adults. In large part, that's because sick children come with anxious parents. Then there were the weekends. For one entire weekend every month, I was on call. That meant I went to work dark and early on Saturday morning and didn't step out into the fresh air until six the following Monday evening.

In 1980, the pediatric cardiology service at the Hospital for Sick Children moved into the newly built wards 4A and 4B. Coincidentally, I began my first year of residency at the hospital in July 1980 and, for my first rotation, was assigned to 4B. My senior resident was Dr. George Rutherford III, who has had a long and distinguished career as a specialist in pediatrics and public health. Currently, he is director of the Institute for Global Health and head of the Division of Preventive Medicine and Public Health at the University of California, San Francisco.

Educated at Stanford University and the Duke University School of Medicine, Rutherford had come to Sick Kids, known then as one of the top five pediatric hospitals in the world, to round out his

American training with "international" experience. Rutherford was not only brilliant, he was also wise in the ways of the world and of residents. The fact that he had been a collegiate teammate of famed tennis player and eight Grand Slam titles winner Jimmy Connors gave me a man-crush on the guy.

Rutherford was adept at sizing up an infant or child who was sick. More than that, he took it upon himself to teach me how to survive as a resident at Sick Kids. Following my first night on call, Rutherford arrived on the ward, saw my haggard appearance, not to mention the deer-in-the-headlights look in my eyes, and made a beeline for me.

"So, Brian," he said, putting a reassuring hand on my shoulder, "how many babies did you box last night?" *Box*, as in coffin. He wanted to know how many patients I'd killed! For a half-second, he kept a perfectly deadpan look on his face, and then broke into a wide grin.

By the time I finished medical school, I'd learned about 20,000 technical terms that laypeople don't know—everything from *aphasia* (the inability to understand language or speak it, a key symptom of stroke) to *zygoma* (the cheekbone). Boxing a patient wasn't among them. Once I got over my initial shock, I was delighted. I have to admit that I found Rutherford's jibe witty and darkly funny. I was quite nervous that first night on call, and Rutherford's slang use of *box* told me that I wasn't alone in that feeling. Moreover, by using it he was letting me into a secret fraternity. It made me want to learn more, as did most of my contemporaries and tens of thousands of young doctors and other health professionals who have followed in our footsteps.

One man who carried his passion for medical slang to another level is Dr. Peter Kussin, respirologist and critical-care physician at Duke University Hospital in Durham, North Carolina. Kussin, a teacher who majored in linguistics and comparative literature before becoming a doctor, is Duke University's resident expert in medical slang. Kussin must love slang, because he picked an awfully strange place to use it. Duke University is well south of the Mason-Dixon Line. It has a buttoned-down, genteel vibe in which slang is considered déclassé and part of gutter culture. That makes Kussin, who was born and raised in New York City and went to medical school there before coming to Duke to do his residency training in the 1980s, an uncomfortable presence.

"The fact that you may have heard that I use and am an aficionado of slang is probably a 70–30 proposition," Kussin said when I visited him in the doctors' lounge at Duke University Hospital—a cavernous, mall-sized room with tall windows and dotted with tables, booths and a cappuccino bar that make it look more like a restaurant than a lounge. Kussin, ever the outsider, eschews the shirts and ties worn by his Deep South colleagues. Bald, rumpled and dressed in comfortable slacks and a blue scrub-suit shirt, the middle-aged internist has a voice that sounds warm, worldly wise and lived-in.

"Seventy percent a compliment and 30 percent wild man," Kussin said, taking note of his reputation as a purveyor of medical argot. "New Yorkers are like that; that's how we roll. We're direct people. That is how you live in a city of 12 million people, right?"

The question was rhetorical. Kussin was the one schooling me in how he came to be a modern-day master of slang. His interest began in the early 1980s, when Kussin was a resident in internal medicine at what was then called Mount Sinai School of Medicine in New York City. The hospital had an *Upstairs, Downstairs* feel to it. One entrance, used by religious Jews, was on Fifth Avenue; the other—used by residents of East Harlem—was on Madison Avenue. The medical students and the residents who trained there were as heterogeneous as the patients. Kussin recalled how medical argot was shared among fellow trainees.

"Medical students weren't allowed to speak it on rounds," he said. "We were not initiated, but amongst ourselves there was a great prize in learning the lingo and then in listening to it and then, in private, using it amongst ourselves."

Lingo such as FLK, which once signified a "funny-looking kid," code for an infant or child born with the visible facial characteristics of a genetic or congenital anomaly such as Trisomy 21, or Down syndrome. Kussin said he recalls being admonished by the chairman of the department of pediatrics at Mount Sinai School of Medicine never to write the letters FLK in a child's hospital chart because the term was insulting and pejorative. What Kussin remembers most about that lecture was that he and his young colleagues ignored it.

"No one was going to pay attention to that," said Kussin. "Our notes, our handovers, our communication—the way we talked to each other—were replete with slang. It was totally politically incorrect—culturally and socioeconomically insensitive—and it was beautiful."

What made it beautiful, he said, was the way slang could tightly pack a lot of telling information about a patient. "It was an era when it was more important to communicate precisely," said Kussin. "When we talked about handoffs, there was nothing better than a handoff done in concise medical slang. There's nothing better than to refer to an obese patient with liver cirrhosis as a Yellow Submarine. They require huge amounts of work and the team has to keep on top of so many things. When you stand in the elevator with one of your buddies and say, 'Yeah, I got this Yellow Submarine,' the person automatically knows what you're talking about, what the problems are and what your mood is because of that."

What Rutherford taught me and what Kussin has taught many others is something called the hidden curriculum of medicine. The phrase *hidden curriculum* comes from a 1968 book by Philip Jackson, *Life in Classrooms*. Jackson observed the behaviour of students in grade-school classrooms. He found that students learned and processed not just academic information in class but social concepts such as co-operating, showing allegiance to both classmates and teachers, and being courteous—and that these traits were essential to getting through school.

Later, in 1970, Benson Snyder, at the time the dean of Institute Relations at the Massachusetts Institute of Technology in Cambridge, Massachusetts, wrote a book titled *The Hidden Curriculum*. In it, Snyder elaborated on a complex array of unstated or hidden academic and social norms and expectations that lead to student anxiety and frustrate students' attempts to think independently. He labelled these items as hidden because they were not set down in course manuals and textbooks, yet were widely known by students to be essential to passing a course and succeeding on campus.

Simply put, the hidden curriculum is the gap between what teachers teach and what students learn. When it comes to studying to be a physician, it turns out there's a lot of curriculum that's hidden.

Dr. Frederic Hafferty, director of the Program in Professionalism and Ethics at the Mayo Clinic in Rochester, Minnesota, is credited as the first academic to identify the hidden curriculum of medicine. In a book chapter titled "The Hidden Curriculum, Structural Disconnects, and the Socialization of New Professionals," Hafferty and co-author Janet Hafler write that the hidden curriculum in medicine "refers to cultural mores that are transmitted, but not openly acknowledged, through formal and informal educational practices."

An outsider with a background in medical sociology and behavioural sciences, Hafferty has spent his entire career studying how medical students and residents learn to be physicians. He began his career in the 1980s, just as medical schools started teaching students about the emerging field of medical ethics. One day, he went to a conference in which speaker after speaker went up to the podium to demand more ethics training for students.

"I just sat in the audience and I thought that this is crazy," Hafferty recalls. "You can give them eighteen courses but there's all kinds of other stuff going on in the environment in medical education that says this stuff is really not all that important compared to all this other stuff you've got to know."

Stuff like knowing where doctors fit in the pecking order of health professionals.

"There are no courses that I know of at medical schools that teach formally that MDs are the best, and everybody else is stupid," says Hafferty. "I can't go into any course catalogue that says MDs are the smartest of the bunch." But physicians learn to think they are.

There also is no course that teaches specialists that they're smarter than family doctors. There's no seminar that trains internists to think surgeons are all do and no think, just as there's no book that teaches surgeons to believe the exact opposite of internists.

The very notion of one group of doctors dissing another may seem odd or even disconcerting to you but, as you'll learn in *The Secret Language of Doctors*, it's woven into the fabric of medicine's culture.

If you want to learn about the ruthlessly competitive streak possessed by many physicians, then mastering the secret language of doctors is essential, says Hafferty: "There's all kinds of stuff that nobody would ever dare put on the books. If you put it on the books, there'd be outrage. So how do you teach it when you can't formally announce that you're teaching it? One of the ways is argot."

A medical textbook or a page on the official website of a hospital might tell me that the orthopedic ward is where patients go to have their hips and knees replaced. But it won't tell me—as some residents have—that the orthopedic ward is sometimes ruefully referred to as being "where patients with diabetes go to die." The acronym FOOBA says basically the same thing—only quicker and more efficiently.

Is that information worth knowing? If, as Hafferty argues, terms such as FOOBA are accurate, they are invaluable to medical practitioners. If you're an internist or resident on call, FOOBA tells you not to walk but to run when you get a call from the orthopedic floor to see a patient in distress. And maybe, if you're a patient or a patient's loved one, knowing about FOOBA tells you to find another hospital.

In a 1998 article titled "Beyond Curriculum Reform: Confronting Medicine's Hidden Curriculum," Hafferty wrote that the hidden curriculum is passed from student to student and from resident to resident not in the classroom but "outside formally identified learning environments: in the elevator, the corridor, the lounge, the cafeteria, or the on-call room."

The Bunker is a compelling way to describe the place where medical students, residents and their attending physicians meet to discuss their patients. Dr. Abraham Verghese is a noted physician and author of the novel *Cutting for Stone*, the *New York Times* medical bestseller set in pre-revolutionary Ethiopia and in a poorly funded New York City hospital. In a 2008 *New England Journal of Medicine* article, "Culture Shock—Patient as Icon, Icon as Patient," Verghese referred to the team room as "a snug bunker filled with glowing monitors." In his article, he encouraged his young charges to abandon the Bunker and spend more time at bedside.

The Bunker also has a much darker meaning. As a twentieth-century cultural reference, the phrase invokes the memory of the *Führerbunker*, a subterranean air-raid shelter near the Reich Chancellery in Berlin that served as the final headquarters of the Third Reich. *The Bunker* is also the title of a 1981 CBS television movie about the last days of the Third Reich, starring Anthony Hopkins, who won an Emmy for his portrayal of Adolf Hitler. In this context, a bunker is a refuge under siege. It may or may not be an accident that *bunker* rhymes with *hunker*, as in "to hunker down."

In the world of hospital medicine, the Bunker is a place where physicians gather strength and find respite amidst a siege of patients and their families. It suggests that physicians—especially young ones—are on a war footing. To extend the analogy, during the Second World War, the Nazis used the Enigma machine to encrypt and decrypt secret messages. Similarly, residents encode their "messages" to keep them from the prying ears of laypeople.

"The Bunker is something I hate," says Dr. Peter Kussin. "I also call it the 'nuclear plant control room.' The Bunker is the place where the residents retreat to avoid going to the bedside. To me it is the place where residents go to avoid nurses, avoid patient contact and avoid hearing bad news. So to me, it is a pejorative."

Dr. Nathan Stall, a first-year resident in internal medicine, budding geriatrician and one of the most thoughtful young minds you'll encounter in the world of medicine, says there is a huge disconnect between what goes on behind the closed doors of the Bunker and what happens when staff interact with patients and their families. "There is that dynamic of what gets talked about in there, the language and the jokes that go on behind the patients' backs."

Being *discharged up*—as opposed to being discharged from hospital—is a casual and flip way of saying a patient has died. Stall remembers the first time he heard it. "I was a naive medical student," he recalls. "I didn't even really know what handover or morning report was. The resident kind of chuckled and said, 'You know, we discharged one up tonight and we're going to discharge two home today.' I turned to the guy and I said, 'What's discharged up?' And he pointed up at the sky."

Discharged up is just one of many euphemisms for death. *Discharged to heaven*, *admitted to the seventeenth floor* (of a hospital with only sixteen floors) and *referred to the outpatient pathology clinic* (pathology being where autopsies are done) are just three other examples. Medical personnel love to craft jests on dark subjects. It's not uncommon for one doctor to tell another that a patient who is dying is "in the departure lounge." We also love puns on common acronyms. Most laypeople know that ICU stands for intensive care unit. In hospital corridors, it's not uncommon to hear about a patient who died on the wards being transferred to the ECU, which is slang for "eternal care unit."

"There was something sort of funny in a dark way about it," says Stall. "You know, there are a lot of laughs and there are often a lot of inappropriate comments made about patients. I don't want to damn the whole profession of internal medicine, but it touches on what really bothers me so much about team medicine and internal medicine."

Stall may be young and idealistic, but he's also right. There is something dark and quite disturbing about the culture of modern medicine that is reflected in the slang used both by young and up-and-coming healers and by their mentors. We're not talking about callous or immoral people. With more than thirty years of practising medicine in my rear-view mirror, I'm still convinced that doctors and other health professionals are among the most ethically grounded people on the planet.

Still, why would young men and women in a caring profession invent and use such language? I put that question to a remarkable group of residents taking postgraduate training at McMaster University's famed Michael G. DeGroote School of Medicine in Hamilton, Ontario. McMaster is one of the most humanistic medical schools on the planet. And yet, even there, young doctors learn and master medical slang.

Dr. Nooreen Popat, a fifth-year resident at McMaster who is training to become a respirologist, told me on *White Coat, Black Art*, the show that I host on CBC Radio One, that getting doctors to admit that they use medical slang is "like admitting to a guilty secret. We all admit that these are terms we're familiar with. None of us really thinks that all of them are appropriate and yet we use them all."

Clarissa Burke, who was finishing a residency in family medicine at McMaster University when I spoke to her on *White Coat, Black Art*, says that "when we use these terms among colleagues, it's one way of really expressing how we feel about a case. You'll have almost instant commiseration from your colleagues because we've almost all been in these situations before. With our colleagues, we understand instantly what it is that they're feeling. There's this instant sort of camaraderie about using terms like that because we all recognize what that person is expressing."

Camaraderie is definitely one reason doctors learn medical slang; it helps us share and process the human tragedies that we witness each and every day we work. Take, for instance, the phrase *peek-and-shriek*, used by surgeons to refer to an operation in which they open up the patient's belly, find it's riddled with cancer and promptly close it up. The slangy rhyme helps fortify them for the long, lonely walk down the hall to the surgical waiting area, where they'll break the worst of all possible news to loved ones gathered to hear something hopeful.

Residents also use slang to complain to their peers about the brutal hours they face as postgraduate trainees. In the past, residents in some specialties (neurosurgery, for example) were expected to work as many as 100 hours a week and as many as thirty-six hours in a row. Concerns about medical errors committed by sleep-deprived residents have led to cutbacks in residents' work schedules. Authorities call the process of giving residents more sleep time "duty hours"—jargon that instantly inspired residents to invent a derisive slang term.

"The one that they came up with was so classic: DOMA—'day off, my ass,'" says Kussin. "They get these days off that really aren't days off because they can't leave the hospital until noon and then they have to be back the next day, so they get like five hours off."

Sometimes, the purpose of slang is to provide a friendly warning to colleagues about a patient. A surgery resident told me that when he's operating on a patient with HIV, it's polite to give everyone in the OR a heads-up so that they can take appropriate precautions to prevent being exposed to the virus—within easy earshot of a patient who may be groggy but still awake. "When I've scrubbed and gone into the operating room, I walk in saying 'double glove' or 'high five,'" says the resident.

Putting on two pairs of gloves is a precaution surgeons take to prevent accidental exposure when they operate on patients with HIV. "High five" is a clever bit of slang that stands for HIV, as in hi-V.

Peter Kussin loves medical argot for another reason: it brings his love of words and letters into the world of clinical medicine. *Yellow Submarine*, for instance, is "very rich and linguistic," says Kussin with a big grin. "It's under the water and it's sort of sinking. It's also a reference to The Beatles' song. It has wit."

But times have changed. The polite reasons that I've listed do not explain why medical slang flourishes nowadays. Other, more sinister factors are at play. Much of today's slang is directed at the growing array of patients that health-care professionals greet with undisguised contempt: the elderly, especially those with dementia; people who refuse to sign a Do Not Resuscitate form when we think it's futile to do CPR; people who are morbidly obese; people with mental health and substance abuse problems; people who are acutely anxious about their health or that of a loved one; and those who come from the economic and social margins of society. Doctors have invented pejorative slang terms for each and every one of these types of patients. Old patients are referred to as FTDs, which stands for "failure to die." Obese patients are called whales. People with borderline personality disorder are called swallowers because sometimes they swallow object like kitchen utensils and nails. People who come often to the ER because they have no other place to receive care are called frequent flyers.

The argot you'll read about in *The Secret Language of Doctors* reduces patients who are ill and in distress to mean-spirited stereotypes. Despite the growing ranks of these patients, the best medical schools in North America continue to crank out class after class of physicians who describe such patients using slang that reveals the utter contempt with which doctors regard them.

We don't like these patients very much—and we like each other even less. Much of the venom spewed in the Bunker is reserved for colleagues. We're supposed to be a team of health professionals, yet we act like a bunch of rabidly competitive and sometimes even bitter rivals.

"Medical training is highly competitive and has historically focused on individual excellence and not necessarily on team building. For many physicians it has been an every-man-for-himself-type workplace," says Dr. Katherine Grichnik, professor of anesthesiology and critical-care medicine in the department of anesthesiology at Duke University Medical Center in Durham, North Carolina. As associate dean for continuing medical education at the Duke School of Medicine, Grichnik is a thought leader in the evolution of professionalism among physicians.

"We're all Type A personalities," she says. "We have fought all our lives to get where we're going. It's always been one test after another, one achievement after another. Then, all of sudden you're at wherever you've achieved or whatever you've thought you were achieving. Once you're in a job or a specialty or a practice, how do you continue to achieve? Well, it's not on test scores anymore. It tends to be more on how can I make myself better? This may be defined differently by different physicians. Luckily for most, the core issue relates to continuing to improve patient care and striving for better outcomes than one's peers.

"Certainly, political and remuneration factors can also come in to play. Clearly, there are appropriate ways to better oneself. And, there are inappropriate ways."

Grichnik is giving her colleagues the benefit of the doubt. From where I sit, a quiet seething goes on inside hospital corridors, a simmering frustration felt by doctors about their work, their patients and each other. It's a low-pitched rumble just below the hearing threshold—enough to irritate and bother my colleagues, even if they don't know why. And the secret language of doctors is flourishing despite the best efforts of medical schools and residency programs to teach young doctors that medical slang is unprofessional and should be eradicated. Like a guilty pleasure, it lives on.

If you or a loved one have entered or are about to enter hospital, *The Secret Language of Doctors* pulls back the curtain to reveal some of medicine's darkest modern secrets. Does your overweight mother's orthopedic surgeon have respect for patients who are obese? Does your heart specialist respect your GP or does she think he is incompetent? Is your dad being transferred to a teaching hospital to help him live or to help him die? This book will give you insight into these and other important questions that you might be reluctant to put into words—let alone ask anyone—insights that are important both for your well-being and for that of the doctors and other health professionals who look after you.

///////

If there's one thing medical sociologist Fred Hafferty wishes, it is to hear first-hand what doctors and other health professionals say when they let their guard down. "I want to be in a room where the conversation is about the hidden curriculum," says Hafferty, "where nobody knows me."

For the past thirty years, I've been in that room. George Rutherford introduced me to medical slang when I was a resident. As a career ER physician who has treated more than 60,000 patients, I've heard the coded words spoken by residents and students and trusted colleagues—and I have experienced the attitudes from which those words were uttered. And now I reveal what I have learned about the culture of medicine to you.

The Secret Language of Doctors is **not** an urban dictionary of medical slang. Many such informal collections of terms can be found on the Internet. To present such a glossary is to imply that all doctors speak slang all the time. I have met many colleagues who never use such terms. More important, in my view, slang is not the problem but the symbolic language that reveals much about what ails medical culture and what needs to be fixed.

I have selected argot that is either typical of many hospitals or particularly revealing about critical aspects of medical culture. My mission is to take you inside the Bunker so that you understand more about our innermost thoughts, attitudes and feelings about modern health care.

Each chapter takes you to a different part of the hospital—from the Emergency Room to the Labor and Delivery floor and from the psychiatry ward to the intensive care unit. I even visited jails and prisons to learn about medical culture in places like those.

In researching the book, I interviewed hundreds of attending physicians, residents, nurses, paramedics and students. In some cases, I have protected their identities. I am grateful to all of them for allowing me to tell their stories in this book.

I have interviewed noted experts in internal medicine, critical care, surgery, obstetrics and gynecology, anesthesiology, nursing and paramedicine. I also interviewed some of the leading thinkers in medical ethics and medical professionalism to find out what they think of medical slang and how they propose to eradicate it. And I tapped into the expertise of some of the world's best and brightest medical sociologists—especially those who have unpacked the hidden curriculum.

Some of the source material for the book comes from interviews that I did for *White Coat, Black Art*. Quotes that are taken from interviews that aired on the show are acknowledged as such. Portions of interviews used in the book that did not air on the program are not acknowledged. In some cases, I conducted interviews intended originally as source material for the book and subsequently used excerpts of these interviews on the show. Again, in such instances, *White Coat, Black Art* is not acknowledged as the original source for the interview.

To protect patient confidentiality, identifying details have been limited or altered. In some cases, patient stories are composites. My first book—*The Night Shift: Real Life in the Heart of the ER*—depicted a typical night shift in the emergency department at Toronto's Mount Sinai Hospital—where I have worked for over twenty-five years. *The Secret Language of Doctors* is not about what goes on at Mount Sinai Hospital but rather about what goes on in hospitals across North America.

As a reader of this book, you may come to know what your doctor really thinks about what's wrong with you, your personality, even your chances of making it out of the hospital alive. *The Secret Language of Doctors* is also a book filled with extraordinary stories of doctors who battle personal and professional obstacles and demons while working to save patients beset by illness and injury. Many of the stories will make you laugh. Some will make you cry. Others will make you angry. However you feel, the next time you find yourself in a hospital elevator with a group of doctors, you'll keep your ears pricked.

But first, let me take you to meet the Harvard-trained physician whose megahit novel introduced generations of young MDs to the world of medical slang and made it cool to speak it.

CHAPTER TWO

Slangmeister

W hen it comes to modern medical slang, there's Before Shem and After Shem. Shem refers to Samuel Shem, the pen name of Dr. Stephen Bergman, psychiatrist and author of the blockbuster novel *The House of God*, which introduced millions of readers—and generations of doctors—to the argot that is the lingua franca of residents and interns then and now. I call Bergman the Slangmeister because until he arrived on the scene in 1978 with his satirical novel, little had been published about medical slang.

The House of God gave the public the first insider's look at the underbelly of hospital life, revealing the hazing, abuse and psychological damage inflicted on medical interns back then and introducing the public and generations of doctors—especially young ones—to a jarringly new kind of medical slang. In doing so, Bergman shook the culture of modern medicine to its very foundation.

By far the most important argot to come from *The House of God* is the term GOMER—an acronym for "get out of my emergency room." In his book, Bergman describes a GOMER as a patient who is frequently admitted to hospital with "complicated but uninspiring and incurable conditions." It's unlikely there's a doctor who has graduated since *The House of God* was published who hasn't heard

GOMER used in that context.

And there are lots more where that came from. *Turf* is a verb that appears frequently in the novel; it refers to finding any excuse to refer a patient to a different department or team. *Buffing* a patient means sorting out medical problems like dehydration before trying to turf. *Bounced* is slang for when a patient who has been turfed is returned to the department or team that turfed her in the first place. *Turf* and *bounce* are used everyday in hospitals across North America; I hear residents at the hospital where I work use them all the time.

Bergman not only introduced those terms, he also acted as a purveyor and catalyst of modern medical slang. Generations of doctors have been influenced and instructed—some might say infected—by Bergman's work. Many of the terms invented since his book was published have their roots in his original slang.

My visit with Bergman in October 2012 at his home in Newton, Massachusetts, a picturesque patchwork of thirteen villages eleven kilometres west of Boston, was like going on an archeological dig through slang history. Bergman and his partner, Janet Surrey, live in a rambling brick building bordered by an old stone fence and with an even older gnarly tree in front. I entered through a back door into a massive white kitchen, where I found Bergman standing beside a large rectangular table, peeling and eating a grapefruit with gusto.

Bergman shook my hand with a strong grip. He looked a bit older than his publicity photos—as if he's gotten leaner as he approaches the end of his seventh decade of life. He appeared comfortable in jeans and a charcoal grey, round-necked T-shirt. He has lost almost all of his hair on top. He had longish hair on the sides and a neatly trimmed beard—both of which were nearly white. Bergman's expression was kind and peaceful. He seemed at ease inside his own skin.

"Have you got a good agent!" Bergman exclaimed almost as soon as we shook hands. He said he'd had lousy agents over the years. As proof, he said that numerous publishers rejected *The House of God* before Richard Marek/Putnam published it. Despite an uncertain beginning, the book has been in print continuously ever since.

I first heard about *The House of God* during my final year of medical school in 1979, just a year after it was published. When my senior resident, George Rutherford III, asked how many patients I'd "boxed" on my first night on call on the cardiology floor at the Hospital for Sick Children, the year was 1980, just two years after *The House of God* was published. Rutherford mentioned the book by name, which made me want to read it. Meanwhile, more and more fellow residents read the book and were starting to quote from it.

After finishing his grapefruit, Bergman—born Jewish but now a practising Buddhist—led me out the back door into the garden and along a path that led to an old two-storey carriage house at the back. He took me up a narrow wooden staircase to a large attic, where he has his office. He sat at a large rectangular desk; behind him, shelf after shelf was crammed with books.

I felt as if I were meeting the proverbial man behind the curtain. I was in the presence of the Wizard: the Great and Powerful Doctor of Medical Words. I asked him many things, but what I wanted to know most of all was where he got the vivid slang he used in *The House of God*. How many of the words were taught to him in medical school and internship? After all, if generations of interns and residents read *The House of God* and learned slang like *turfing* and *bouncing* from Bergman, then Bergman must have borrowed argot he heard on the hospital wards in much the same way. Bergman's answer was startling.

"Well, I don't think actually any of them were taught to me when I was a medical student," he said. But when he started his internship at Beth Israel Hospital in Boston in 1973–74, "GOMER was in use. I didn't invent that. I did invent GOMERE (pronounced "go-mare"), which is the female. Either I invented most of the others in the novel when I was writing it or I did so joking around with some guys. I can't remember now which is which, but *buff* and *turf*, I think that was sort of a group thing that evolved. I'm sure I thought of the *bounce*. The thing is, it's one thing to have this language. I codified it. I took it further."

///////

Bergman took a nascent secret language and made it deeper and broader than ever before. Until *The House of God*, almost nothing had been published on medical slang or on the culture of medicine from which it came.

One of the closest I found was an article published in 1973 in the journal *American Speech* by Philip C. Kolin, an American author, poet and currently a University Distinguished Professor in the College of Arts and Letters and professor of English at the University of Southern Mississippi in Hattiesburg. In an article titled "The Language of Nursing," Kolin noted the growing number of medical dramas on television—such as *Medical Center, Marcus Welby, M.D.* and *M*A*S*H*—that were being "eagerly received by the viewing public." Kolin—an outsider to the world of medicine—was the first to observe there was something more to the language than efficient communication of highly specialized information. He noted that nurses used dignified language when speaking to patients but exercised less caution in collegial conversation. Kolin wrote that a hospital gown is sometimes referred to as a "monkey jacket," and that "chandelier syndrome" refers to the tendency of a patient startled by the coldness of a stethoscope on the skin to jump toward the ceiling.

I can remember hearing a variation of that phrase during my training. We called it "the chandelier sign." More than one attending or resident gynecologist taught me that a doctor could diagnose a woman with pelvic inflammatory disease (PID) by demonstrating that her cervix was tender to touch and therefore inflamed. As he explained it, the way to determine if a cervix is tender is to don a lubricated glove and wiggle the woman's cervix from side to side. The official name of this finding is cervical motion tenderness. The slang phrase made me cringe then, and still does.

In Kolin's article, patients with alcohol dependence were called alkies. Those with drug addiction were labelled ads. Nurses called patients with manic depression (now called bipolar affective disorder) manics, and referred to those with schizophrenia as schizzes. Commonly, they described patients agitated by psychiatric disorders as bouncing off the walls; such patients were placed in a quiet room, or QR, until their agitation settled. Such slang terms tell me that non-psychiatric health professionals back then were as mystified and threatened by emotionally disturbed patients as we are today. The only thing that has changed is that it's no longer considered politically correct to use such terms.

Kolin also discovered a nickname for what was then called electric shock treatment (EST). He wrote: "When, as frequently occurs, their doctors order an EST 'electric shock treatment,' the nursing staff say they are going to zap a patient." Today, EST is known as electroconvulsive therapy (ECT). It is a psychiatric treatment that induces a seizure in an anesthetized patient for therapeutic benefit. Although considered controversial by some, ECT is recognized as a valid treatment for severe depression that hasn't responded to antidepressants and other therapies, as well as for mania and catatonia.

What surprises me about the use of the slang verb *to zap* a patient is its wider cultural context. Ken Kesey's novel *One Flew Over the Cuckoo's Nest*—set in an Oregon psychiatric hospital and featuring graphically disturbing descriptions of patients receiving ECT— had been around for eleven years by then and even adapted into a

Broadway play. Just two years following the publication of Kolin's article, an Academy Award-winning film version of the novel was released.

The early twentieth century brought the first references to modern medical slang. A 1927 article, "Hospital Talk," by Dorothy Barkley, published in the journal *American Speech*, introduced phrases such as *scrub nurse* and *scrub room* to the public. But Barkley also captured some pointedly unflattering terms. "A woman physician invading a profession dominated by men," wrote Barkley, "is a hen-medic, and, in many minds, is schizy to do such a thing. [*Schizy*], culled from the term schizophrenia, means much the same as the colloquial crazy."

Dorothy House, in her 1938 article "Hospital Lingo," also published in *American Speech*, was one of the first to identify a hierarchy of medical trainees. She wrote that although they were both medical school graduates studying at a hospital, residents outranked interns by reason of experience. Often, interns were known as house men. She wrote that the newest intern "may be assigned to routine laboratory tests and called a pup or junior." Today, we call them *scut dogs*—*scut work* referring to the endless paperwork and other tasks that residents consider beneath them.

House wrote that patients who were critically ill and near death were on something called the DL, or danger list. I've heard of DL signifying keeping things on the down low or referring to a baseball team's disabled list, but I've never heard that use of DL in medical circles.

In a 1961 article, Peter Hukill and James Jackson wrote about "an extensive, informal language" they referred to as argot, slang or cant. Much of it was technical. An electrocardiogram was shortened into an ECG or EKG, an intravenous into an IV and morphine sulfate into MS. A *lunger* was a patient with a chronic lung disease such as emphysema or tuberculosis, and a *stroker* a patient with a stroke. Hukill and James wrote that the word *terminal* was used to describe a patient approaching death, but it is passé these days because lay-people know what it means. But the jargon term *pre-terminal*—as in pre-terminal cancer—is still used widely.

Hukill and James cited two examples of pejorative argot. *Out in left field* was slang for a patient who is disoriented or out of touch with reality, a phrase still used by health professionals. The most astonishing piece of slang on the list is *crock*, which the authors defined as "a patient who complains continually of multiple symptoms, many of which are either imaginary or of psychic origin; one whose complaints are out of proportion to his illness." I've been hearing patients described as crocks since I was a medical student.

But those were sporadic examples. For medical slang as reflected in the novel by Bergman and in the academic writings of Kolin to take off, some wholesale changes in the culture of modern medicine had to occur.

The era after the Second World War brought incredible transformations to health care. Surgeons carried out the first successful heart, lung and liver transplants. Vaccines for measles and rubella were developed. Birth control pills and the intrauterine device ushered in an era of sexual freedom. In 1964, the U.S. Surgeon General first linked cigarette smoking to lung cancer, emphysema and heart disease.

But amidst the awe and wonder of new medical discoveries, a growing cynicism was bubbling just under the surface of medical culture. Thalidomide, an anti-nausea and sedative drug, was introduced as a sleeping pill in the late 1950s; doctors began to prescribe it to pregnant women for morning sickness. The drug was withdrawn after numerous reports of catastrophic birth defects. Advocates for victims of thalidomide say the drug affected more than 10,000 babies worldwide. Canada has the dubious distinction of being the last country in the world to pull thalidomide from pharmacy shelves.

The drug was never approved for use in the United States. However, there are twenty-six known American thalidomide victims. Although the Food and Drug Administration was lauded for keeping thalidomide off American pharmacy shelves, the experience in other countries led to tougher regulatory standards. The lasting legacy of this episode was that it underscored the capability of pharmaceutical drugs and other "wonders of modern medicine" to do great harm—a lesson that would be repeated again and again in the decades to follow.

The 1960s and '70s also brought tumultuous changes to the health system. Canada introduced universal health care in 1966, and health care became the fastest growing industry in the United States in the '60s. Doctors went from seeing themselves mainly as healers and maintainers of their patients' health to running their practices like businesses. As you'll see, these developments put in place some of the conditions that made medical slang flourish in the 1980s.

During the '60s the United States experienced a violent political era that included the civil rights movement, the Vietnam War, the assassinations of President John F. Kennedy, his brother Robert F. Kennedy and civil rights leader Dr. Martin Luther King, and the Watergate scandal that led to the resignation of President Richard Nixon in 1974. Bergman was a member of the generation of students that came of age during that time. They believed in the power of protest as a force to correct injustice. Their protests helped end the Vietnam War and helped create civil rights laws.

In July 1973, Stephen Bergman, then a 29-year-old just graduated from Harvard Medical School, began his internship in Boston at what was then called the Beth Israel Hospital. Five years later, writing under the pen name Samuel Shem, Bergman used his experience at Beth Israel as the basis for *The House of God.*

The book was a blockbuster. *The House of God* has sold more than two million copies and has been published in thirty languages. The famed British medical journal *The Lancet* named *The House of God* one of the two most important American medical novels of the twentieth century.

The novel follows Dr. Roy Basch during his year of internship at House of God, which stands in for Beth Israel Hospital (known today as Beth Israel Deaconess Medical Center). Like Bergman, Basch arrives on his first day completely unprepared for the responsibilities and long hours heaped upon him. A wise senior resident, an anti-hero named The Fat Man, befriends him.

The Fat Man teaches Basch to keep his patients alive—and to survive internship—by deliberately disobeying the rules of so-called good patient care set by the hospital and the system in general. He teaches him instead to follow the thirteen subversive laws revealed during the course of the book. My favourite is Law No. 3: "At a cardiac arrest, the first procedure is to take your own pulse." *Cardiac arrest* itself is a medical euphemism for heart stoppage, meaning the patient is clinically dead and in immediate need of resuscitative measures—cardiopulmonary resuscitation (CPR), inserting a breathing tube, defibrillating or shocking the heart, and administering medications to normalize the heart rhythm and raise the blood pressure.

Nowadays, we call it a code—short for Code Blue, the near-universal designation for cardiac arrest. Residents on call carry arrest pagers; when a patient is found in cardiac arrest, a health-care worker or a bystander pushes a big red button (located on the wall near the patient's bed and in patient bathrooms) that automatically pages the cardiac arrest team. Residents on call drop whatever they are doing and run to the patient's bedside. (I remember running half a kilometre across the sprawling Sunnybrook Health Sciences Centre complex, up a staircase to the sixth floor and arriving at the bedside gasping for breath—only to find that the patient himself had pressed the arrest button, thinking it was the nurse call button!)

By the time I read Bergman's book around 1980, I had attended many cardiac arrests and had sometimes reached the patient's bedside feeling so panicky that I wouldn't remember what drugs to order and what voltage to use when shocking the heart. I took The Fat Man's advice and often ran to the patient's bedside with my finger on my own pulse.

No sooner was the ink dry on Bergman's book than residents and interns throughout North America began inventing laws of their own. Around that time, I recall a resident telling me, with a conspiratorial smile, a rather shocking adaptation for pediatrics of one of The Fat Man's laws: "You can't kill a Down's," he said. It was a direct steal of the First Law of *The House of God*: "GOMERs don't die." Down syndrome, also known as Trisomy 21, is caused by the presence of all or part of a third copy of chromosome 21. Down syndrome, named after John Langdon Down, the British doctor who was among the first to describe it, is recognizable by distinctive facial characteristics. It is associated with short stature and reduced cognitive abilities. It can also cause vision and hearing disorders, as well as congenital heart disease, underactive thyroid and certain forms of cancer. Like GOMERs, some kids with Down syndrome have many medical problems and require frequent admissions to hospital.

What the resident was saying is that no matter what the doctor does, these kids keep getting sick but keep surviving, only to get sick again. I took it as a statement of grudging admiration for the durability of children with Down syndrome.

You might find the awful phrase shocking, as I do today. In fairness, you have to remember that the resident used it in 1980. I suspect the doctor would cringe hearing those words from so long ago repeated in a book. But that's not the point. The resident smiled while saying the words, as if emulating The Fat Man introducing me to the facts of medical life. And, as surprised and disturbed as I may have been to hear kids with Down syndrome spoken of in that way, I have to admit that I was glad to be let in on the joke—however distasteful.

/////////

Conversations like the one I had with that pediatric resident have played out in hospital elevators, bunkers, and on-call rooms and at nursing stations across North America and around the world ever since. Fat Men, and perhaps even Fat Women, were repeating the rules and the slang set forth by Stephen Bergman in *The House of God*—and making up many of their own. In 1999, *Newsweek* listed *The House of God* as "*the* novel to read about becoming a doctor."

The House of God has been so influential for several reasons. One can't ignore the fact that Bergman wrote a great book. He had and still has an ear for language and an ability to write the way doctors talk. Bergman's take on the culture of modern medicine at that time—including the hazing of interns and residents and the futility of medical care served up to frail seniors with dementia—sounded authentic, or at least plausible. Interns and residents could see themselves as Roy Basch or The Fat Man.

For decades before Bergman wrote his book, interns and residents battled brutal schedules, sleep deprivation and emotional abuse. What made *The House of God* special was that Bergman was the first to say emphatically that the system was sick and that it was okay for interns and residents to rail against it.

Bergman invented a secret language that helped Basch and his fellow interns cope with their fictional hospital of despair. In so doing, he validated the use of that secret language in everyday conversation in hospitals in the real world. As with a secret handshake, Bergman invited interns and residents to join an exclusive club. And join they did.

More than thirty-five years have passed since *The House of God* was published. In researching *The Secret Language of Doctors*, I interviewed dozens of residents, attending physicians and surgeons, nurses and paramedics. Even today, the slang codified by Stephen Bergman is used, or at the very least known, by all of them.

"Every medical student should read it," said Dr. Todd Raine, a nine-year veteran of emergency medicine at St. Paul's Hospital in Vancouver. "Not as a paragon of what medicine should be, although there are facets of it that I still think ring very true. Some of them—like 'Do as little as humanly possible'—are very true these days, [when] we oversee a lot of stuff we don't have to. Most of us can quote the rules, if not by number at least by knowing what they are."

From 2007 to 2012, Dr. Christian Jones did a residency in general surgery at the University of Kansas Medical Center in Kansas City, Kansas, becoming chief resident in his final year. Nobody's claiming that *The House of God* is a textbook, or even factual, but it's entertaining and teaches you a lot about the jadedness you're going to see, in residency especially," said Jones. "While that may not be something that a lot of people admit is there, it most certainly is. And I don't personally see a problem with getting that first exposure from a book, rather than from being shocked when you start your residency."

What's telling about the state of modern health care is the extent to which medical wannabes have not only embraced the secret language; they have embellished it. Dr. Christopher Kinsella is a resident in general surgery at Saint Louis University Hospital in St. Louis, Missouri, who blogs at scrubsisreal.com. Where he works, they don't turf patients to a different department or team; they *do a lateral.* For the uninitiated, a *lateral* refers to a lateral pass—a term used in American and Canadian football as well as in rugby. The ball carrier—often but not always the quarterback—throws the ball not forward but to a teammate beside or behind him.

"Let's say there's a patient I'm taking care of who is no longer interesting to me," says Kinsella. "They don't need surgery but they're sick. The patient needs to be in a hospital, they need to be taken care of by someone, but they don't need to be taken care of by a surgeon. So we would try to lateral to another ward."

As in football, a patient lateral may be attempted by a doctor who has done all he or she can think of doing to help a patient who isn't responding to treatment. Sometimes, it's done to remove a difficult patient from the doctor's list. "I'm done running with this ball," says Kinsella. "I need to send this to someone else. They can run with the ball now."

Databases are filled with slang words and phrases that make up medical argot. A 1993 paper by Robert Coombs, Sangeeta Chopra, Debra Schenk and Elaine Yutan, published in the journal *Social Science & Medicine,* used what was described as a "sociolinguistic approach" to compile an impressive list of more than 300 slang terms culled from medical personnel and publications about hospital life. Sorry to say, the largest body of slang unearthed by the authors consists of highly unflattering descriptions of patients—especially patients regarded as difficult.

The article defined *toad* as a "troublesome and demanding patient." A *blabber* is a "patient who talks excessively." A *troll* is a "patient who is a big pain in the neck; old, debilitated, and sometimes incontinent." A *Camille,* named for the Alexandre Dumas heroine in *La Dame aux Camélias* who dies dramatically from tuberculosis in her lover's arms, is a "patient who chronically feels about to die and is very vocal about it."

Health professionals love devising acronyms: type 2 diabetes is shortened to DM2, congestive heart failure into CHF, gastroesophageal reflux disease into GERD, and so forth. Coombs and his co-authors discovered that the playful desire to create acronyms carries over into slang. The article describes COP as an acronym for "crotchety old patient," HOWDY as short for "hypertensive obese white diabetic yahoo," and DIAL as short for "dumb in any language." "Informal medical language, neither taught in the classroom nor recorded in textbooks, is no less dynamic in clinical settings," Coombs and his colleagues wrote in 1993.

In July 2011, *Scrubs*, which bills itself as "the leading lifestyle magazine for nurses," published the Top 47 slang terms nurses use, along with suggested usages of the terms. Top of the list: PITA, an acronym for "pain in the ass." Second on the list is BATS, short for "broke all to shit."

All of this medical slang exists in part because *The House of God* made it acceptable, even desirable.

Even critics of medical slang—including Dr. Katherine Grichnik of the Duke University Hospital Medical Center—acknowledge the seminal role played by Stephen Bergman. "*The House of God* was a witty, interesting, amazing book that revealed some medical culture," says Grichnik. "But at the same time I think he propagated a few stereotypes that are just patently false. Medical students read it and, all of a sudden, the meter is set. This is the way medicine is. This is how we should all behave and act—and that's just not true."

/////////

Why did Bergman invent and disseminate a secret language? "We were in a perfect storm of desperation," he said. "The desperate invent slang because what else are you going to do? You've got to kind of laugh and get through it." That rings true—especially if you go back to Victor Hugo's definition of argot as "the language of misery."

Bergman's internship at Beth Israel Hospital amounted to a form of poorly paid servitude. He worked 100-hour weeks and was on call every second night, which meant he had no life outside of work. "The patient load was large. We were incredibly alone with all that we were doing. And we were tired as hell because the hours were awful."

But that can't be the whole story. After all, the hours residents work today aren't nearly as brutal, yet medical slang lives on.

Perhaps it's the psychological abuse by senior physicians that tipped the scales—something Bergman said he experienced at Beth Israel. Bergman attributed this to the rigid hierarchical structure of hospital medicine in which attending physicians lord it over interns and residents. "Like all medical students, residents and other lower-downs, I have been humiliated many times," said Bergman.

But unlike *The House of God*'s Roy Basch, who had a kind mentor, Bergman had no one to teach him how to learn to survive in a hospital in which residents like him—not to mention his patients—were treated inhumanely. "We had nobody," said Bergman. "There was no Fat Man, really. I invented that we had a dude."

Far from having a dude, Bergman recalled that the chief resident he served under was a bootlicker. "The chief resident was an absolute jerk. He had only one thing on his mind, which was to do nothing that would alienate the chief of staff, the other faculty and senior staff so he could get a job at the Beth Israel Hospital and buy his horse farm out in Sudbury [a tony enclave near Boston]."

For Dr. Peter Kussin of Duke University Hospital, the slang found in *The House of God* brought validation, making it okay to infuse medical terminology with a bit of wit. Moreover, Kussin said, Bergman's book provided him with the cover he needed to become a slangmeister himself in the 1980s, without incurring universal disapproval from his buttoned-down colleagues at Duke. "It's good to know that I'm not so much of an anomaly because all the people of my era used slang and spoke slang," said Kussin.

That said, very few have tried to keep it alive as Kussin has. The internist has crisscrossed the United States giving speeches on the language doctors use to converse informally with one another. Had Bergman completed his residency in internal medicine and not become a psychiatrist, Kussin would be his rival as the modern slangmeister.

Like Kussin, I see the current use of slang as a yearning to put back some wit and wordplay into a world of medicine that long ago replaced literature and poetry with a nearly exclusive emphasis on science—much to its detriment.

/////////

Then, as now, the laws of *The House of God* ran counter to the culture of established medicine as taught by Bergman's mentors and mine. According to an article by Bergman (under his pen name Shem) published in 2012 in *The Atlantic,* his book left the medical establishment up in arms. "I was maligned and disliked," wrote Bergman. "The book was censored by medical school deans, who often kept me from speaking at their schools. None of it really bothered me, though. I was secure in the understanding that all I had done was tell the truth about medical training."

As an intern, Bergman absorbed the culture of internal medicine at one of Harvard's famed teaching hospitals and captured it in his book. But he was just passing through. Following his internship, Bergman did a residency in psychiatry at McLean Hospital in Belmont, Massachusetts. Until he retired from medicine to write full-time in 2005, Bergman had a private practice in psychiatry, with an interest in patients with addiction disorders, and was a professor of psychiatry at Harvard Medical School.

Bergman says he never personally experienced the deep sense of humiliation from some quarters of medicine that he depicted in *The House of God*. "I don't get much bothered by fear or humiliation if I know that what I did was authentic and deft," he told me.

But he says he did have just such an experience after he joined Harvard's faculty as a psychiatrist. Years ago, Bergman said, he taught a course in which third-year students were supposed to be able to talk in small groups about difficult experiences they were having as they adjusted from lecture halls to working on hospital wards. "In a group meeting to review the first year of the course, I said I felt that what the students really needed was to talk in safety about their stressful and brutalizing experiences," Bergman recalled. "At that point, a famous surgeon interrupted me and, in front of my colleagues, said: 'What do you want to turn this into—a year-long psychiatric séance?'"

The remark left Bergman speechless. In *The House of God*, a character named Potts becomes depressed and commits suicide and a second character suffers a psychotic break—something that actually happened to one of Bergman's fellow interns at Beth Israel. Both were consequences of the psychological toll inflicted on interns and residents of the 1970s. Bergman felt he was being mocked yet again for raising the issue with his fellow teachers. "I ended my association with teaching at Harvard Medical School," he says.

I wanted to know why Bergman the slangmeister thinks medical argot has thrived in the years since his book was published. "Slang makes a very good connection among all those who share it," he said. "They invent slang, sometimes to distance themselves from patients, sometimes to just amuse themselves, sometimes to break the tension, sometimes to be on the same page, and sometimes to bond."

But it's a bond and a language that can be as insulting to patients as it is jarring. And it's not going away. Bergman may not have a building named after him, but he has a legacy of medical slang and an enduring impact on the culture of modern medicine much more lasting than bricks and mortar.

CHAPTER THREE

Code Brown and Other Bodily Fluids

sk many people why they didn't become doctors and they'll say that they can't stand the sight of blood. Who are they trying to kid? Try feces or vomit or pus so smelly it can make the sturdiest resident faint. How about maggots emerging from a patient's orifices? Now you get what I mean.

Think the health professions are all glory? A lot of the time they're just plain gory.

From early on in our training my colleagues and I get thrown into the proverbial deep end of an effluent pool. We must learn to overcome our own urge to hurl while somehow making it seem to you as if it's just another day at the office.

One of the ways we cope with our own sense of discomfort and even disgust is by trading stories laced with a liberal dose of medical slang. The most universal example is Code Brown.

I've already described the term Code Blue, the very common designation for cardiac arrest requiring a medical team—sometimes called a code team—to rush to the patient's bedside and begin immediate resuscitative efforts. Code Blue is an example of medical argot that was developed as a neutral way to announce on a hospital intercom that a patient is in cardiac arrest and needs help—without frightening visitors and other patients. TV shows including *ER* and *Grey's Anatomy*—eager to make their stories as realistic as possible— have adopted the term. And once that happened, Code Blue entered the public vernacular and ceased being argot.

At my hospital, Code Pink means a newborn is in need of immediate resuscitation. Code Red refers to smoke detected somewhere in the hospital. Code White means a patient is missing. There is no international convention in colour-coding. Different countries use different colours to connote different medical emergencies.

In some hospitals, Code Brown signifies an environmental emergency or one that involves hazardous materials. But it's also known almost universally as slang for a patient poop emergency.

"It's the perfect default label," says Dr. Erin Sullivan, a registered nurse who went back to school at the University of Limerick in Ireland to become a physician. "When you're giving report [at nursing handover], if there's family members around or there's people milling in and out, you're not going to say the patient was shitting himself the whole night long, even if you know that's what was happening. If you say it was a Code Brown, it makes it maybe a little more professional sounding if other ears were to hear it."

As a doctor, my usual relationship with Code Brown is olfactory. I step onto a ward and it hits my nostrils like a dog kennel just after breakfast. I switch to mouth breathing, and head in the opposite direction—testing my nostrils now and then—until the smell is down to an acceptable level. But if you're the nurse looking after the patient who emits the Code Brown, it might well be your professional obligation to run—not away from the scene but right toward its smelly epicentre.

I see Code Browns, but other than changing my kids' dirty diapers, I have never had to clean one up. But nurses do, and that's why they remember Code Brown patients in pungently nauseating detail. One nurse told me about a patient who kept soiling himself throughout an entire shift. "He was about 400 pounds," the nurse recalls. "He couldn't move at all, even from side to side. He just had constant diarrhea. It was unrelenting. At nighttime, there was only one other nurse in the department, so it was my job the entire twelve-hour shift to try and turn him as much as I could, pull the sheet out, put a new sheet down, turn him on the other side, pull the old sheet out, pull the new one across. Then the process would just start over again." The nurse says she remembers getting through the experience with "a lot of sweating and cussing."

Doctors refer to a loss of bowel control as fecal incontinence. A study published in 1995 in the *Journal of the American Medical Association* pegged the prevalence of fecal incontinence at 2 to 3 percent. There are many reasons for fecal incontinence. Some people are born with it. Bowel diseases such as Crohn's, anal surgery and even trivial anal conditions such as hemorrhoids can cause it. A vaginal birth—the most common cause of incontinence in young and otherwise healthy women—can damage the anal sphincter or the nerve that controls it. Medical conditions such as diabetes, stroke, even a slipped disc can damage the sphincter's nerve supply.

The vast majority of patients who inspire Code Brown stories are elderly—and it's more common in women than in men. Older patients often have a condition called sigmoid volvulus, an intestinal disorder in which the lower part of the large intestines called the sigmoid colon gets blocked. The way to unblock the sigmoid colon is to insert a short endoscope called a sigmoidoscope through the anus; once the scope is in place, the doctor inserts a long plastic rectal tube about the diameter of a garden hose through the scope and into the intestine until it reaches the blockage. The tube becomes the conduit through which trapped poop and gas are expelled.

This procedure is invasive enough that most nurses are not permitted to do it. If you're the doctor inserting the tube, the most important thing a thoughtful mentor teaches you is to stand as far away as you can from the end of the tube protruding from the anus—to avoid the nearly inevitable mess that ensues when the intestine stuffed with feces and gas is rather suddenly decompressed.

Dr. Nathan Stall, a resident in internal medicine, knows what's at stake. The first time he tried to insert a tube, a more senior resident was watching. "The rookie mistake is to not connect the rectal tube to the bag," says Stall. "The senior was raising his hand to warn me but it was too late. There was like a 'ping,' and the stool shot across the room and hit the curtain. The senior resident actually had to jump out of the way so as to not be hit with this high-velocity stool flying across the room. It was hysterical to us, but you have to try and maintain some professionalism. I'll never forget to connect the bag to the rectal tube should I ever have to do that again."

One mentor who is kind enough to put his young charges in the know is Dr. Marcus Burnstein, a veteran colorectal surgeon at St. Michael's Hospital in Toronto. "The old joke in medical school or in general surgical residency is that when you find a patient in the emergency department with a sigmoid volvulus who needs this procedure, it's the perfect opportunity to bring the third-year medical student down and get him or her to do it to see if they can get outta the way fast enough," says Burnstein.

"In the intensive care unit (ICU), when we had a Code Brown, everybody would go in, gown up and put masks on," says Megen Duffy, an American ER nurse who blogs as Not Nurse Ratched, a reference to the cold, heartless nurse in *One Flew Over the Cuckoo's Nest*.

Duffy remembers a particularly gruesome Code Brown on a patient admitted to the cardiac ICU. The patient had *Clostridium difficile* (we call it *C. diff*), a hospital superbug that has been linked to deadly outbreaks. It's a potentially life-threatening intestinal infection that causes profuse, foul-smelling diarrhea. "I spent the entire night putting on gown and gloves to go in there and clean up his stool and wash his hands with soap and water, because that's the only thing that kills *C. diff*, and hang antibiotics and hang his feedings and clean around his Foley [catheter]," recalls Duffy. "By the time I did all that and took off my gown and went and took care of my other patient, it was time to go back in there. I think I went through fifty of those isolation gowns. It was awful."

For some residents, the fact that Code Brown is usually the nurses' problem gives them an outlet for *schadenfreude*—enjoyment in seeing the troubles of others. "I've seen residents chuckle when the nurse who has been giving them a hard time or paging them for things that probably they didn't need to be bothered for has to go clean that up," says Duffy.

Paramedics have their share of dealing with Code Brown emergencies too. Morgan Jones Phillips, a nine-year veteran paramedic with Emergency Medical Services in Toronto, won the *NOW* Audience Choice Award at Toronto's SummerWorks Theatre Festival in 2008 with his first solo play, *The Emergency Monologues,* a series of stories inspired by his career as a paramedic.

"This is kind of mean, but it's always a little bit satisfying when it happens to the fancy people that go clubbing downtown," says Phillips. "They're all dressed up super nice and fancy. Guys have shaved their chests and they're all super ready to score. But then they have poo running down their legs. There's a special horror that comes when a woman poos while wearing nylons."

The horror is even greater when a Code Brown happens in the back of the ambulance. "It happens lots of times while driving that the patient—especially if they come in with stomach flu or they come in with diarrhea or tarry stool [also known as melena, a thick, oozy, formless bowel movement whose black, tarry consistency is caused by gastrointestinal bleeding]. If we think they're about to have diarrhea or they say they think it's going to happen again, we flick the lights on and try and get to the hospital as fast as we can."

I don't blame paramedics one bit for trying to get Code Brown patients to the hospital as quickly as possible. If the patient defecates in the back of the ambulance, it's the job of the paramedics to clean it up.

⁄⁄⁄⁄⁄⁄⁄

If you have to endure a Code Brown experience, there is at least one compensation: you have a good story to tell colleagues.

Marc Burnstein says telling Code Brown stories is a way colleagues bond. "It's that dark humour," he says. "If we tell each other stories and have a little laugh about it, maybe it takes away some of the unpleasantness."

Scrubsmag.com, which bills itself as "the nurses' guide to good living," has pages of posts filled with Code Brown stories. Here is one from 2012 by a registered nurse named Amy Mickschl; she remembers one patient who produced loose stool almost continuously: "I was changing her soiled bed one night and was just getting ready to put a new brief on . . . when she coughed and sprayed diarrhea all over the bed, wall and me. Thank god it didn't hit me in the face!"

Mickschl goes on to describe home remedies to deal with the smell—sucking on cinnamon-flavoured Altoids, putting a dab of Vicks VapoRub under the nose, even wearing two surgical masks with a squirt of toothpaste on the inside—anything to counteract an aroma that can be overwhelming.

Talking about that Code Brown with colleagues the next morning was all about a different sort of code—giving fellow nurses on the day shift a heads-up about what duties lay ahead. "The nurses knew which patient I had been working with the night before," writes Mickschl, "so, of course, the next thing that happens is that everyone's arguing over who has to take that patient that day. No one wants that patient that day. It's like, oh, god, you would do anything not to have that patient."

Imagine for a moment the chilly reception Mickschl would have received from the nurse on the day shift who ended up caring for the woman with diarrhea if Mickschl hadn't given her a heads-up.

For nurses like Amy Mickschl and paramedics like Morgan Phillips, these shared stories speak to the powerlessness they feel about having to do a clean-up job most of us would rather avoid.

But even that is changing. "Are Student Nurses Too Posh To Wash?" asked the provocative headline on an article published in 2009 on nursingtimes.net. Author Gabriel Fleming quoted a nursing student who was reported to have told a staff nurse: "I keep being asked to do things which won't help me learn—clear up poo, mop up blood, give patients tea and toast. I realized that I needed to be more focused to learn, and I don't do those sorts of things now."

Laura Servage believes this attitude is part of a larger phenomenon. Servage is a PhD candidate at the University of Alberta who focuses on educational policy studies, as well as on learning, training and the impact of post-secondary education on society. She writes a blog titled *My So-Called Career*. In a post from March 2010 titled "All About Bedpans: How Credentials Stratify Work," Servage argued persuasively that as nurses aspire to higher education and higher professional credentials (something she referred to in her blog as credentialization), some—like the nursing student in Gabriel Fleming's article—may think differently about the meaning of their work.

"It's not a frivolous question," wrote Servage. "What I'm thinking about here is something akin to an unrecognized caste system, which is entrenched both through professionalization and, in many cases, unionization. Basically, the more thoroughly we are able to describe work—name positions and place boundaries around the nature of tasks that will and will not be performed—the more opportunity there is to segregate 'good work' from 'not so good work.'"

Nowadays, there are several different castes (as Servage put it) of nurses. A registered nurse (RN) in the U.S. or Canada is a graduate of a nursing program at a post-secondary institution who has passed a national licensing exam. One level below the RN is a licensed practical nurse (LPN), the term used in both countries for a nurse trained at a vocational or technical school or a community college. LPNs care for patients under the direction of physicians and registered nurses. They take vital signs, prepare and give injections, keep patients comfortable and assist with bathing, dressing and personal hygiene.

One level above RN is a nurse practitioner (NP). This is an advanced-practice registered nurse who has completed a graduate degree (a master's or doctorate). Unlike RNs and LPNs, NPs have an enhanced scope of practice that permits them to make certain types of diagnoses, order tests and start treatment. Because they have a scope of practice independent of physicians, NPs are permitted to see and treat patients on their own.

It certainly makes one wonder just which of those three types of nurses have the task of changing bedpans. None of them, says Servage—not even the LPNs. "It is not the licensed practical nurse's job to clean bedpans anymore."

It turns out the system has created a whole new type of health-care worker to do the job: the nursing assistant. Nursing assistants help patients with physical, mental and cognitive impairments with health-care needs that include activities of daily living. "They do the heavy lifting and change the bedpans," says Servage.

And what about the nurses? "They want to do the more intellectual work that comes with nursing," she says.

This thinking isn't just going on inside the minds of individual nurses; Servage argues it's happening at the professional and union levels as well. "If occupations have different status, then there's all sorts of incentives to make your job not the job of emptying bedpans." Servage worries who will be left to do that job—and how well they'll be trained to do it. "How many layers of professions can we have before we hit the wall? Who is cleaning the bedpans? Who is taking the vocational courses to work in health care?"

This is no idle concern. In Canada in 2011, the Cape Breton District Health Authority in Nova Scotia had an outbreak of *C. difficile*; thirty-two of forty-one cases were hospital-acquired. A factor in the outbreak was the improper cleaning of bedpans: hospital personnel cleaned bedpans in patient bathrooms rather than in separate utility rooms.

One professional who shows no reluctance to clean up Code Browns is Nicole Donaldson, a licensed practical nurse in British Columbia. She says she hates it when registered nurses she works with don't feel the same way. "I had a lady who had cancer and the RN who was trying to change her colostomy was retching," Donaldson recalls. "The poor woman was absolutely sobbing uncontrollably because this nurse was making such a theatrical fuss about the smell. I really felt sorry for that lady and I think from that day forward I always thought to myself, 'If you can't do it, then you get somebody in that can do it.'"

So far, I've told you stories about Code Browns as recounted by the doctors who witness them and the nurses, nurse assistants and paramedics who clean them up. What's missing is the perspective of the person most affected by a Code Brown: the patient. That Nicole Donaldson even thinks about the patient in the midst of a Code

Brown is exceptional. What's striking about Code Brown stories is that they usually ignore the patient's point of view. It's almost as if we blame patients for pooping uncontrollably—as if they wouldn't do almost anything to avoid it.

Just ask Sholom Glouberman, a health policy insider who experienced an embarrassing episode of fecal incontinence several years ago. After his surgeon removed a non-cancerous polyp from his large intestine, a post-operative infection nearly cost Glouberman his life. As a result, he co-founded a national organization dedicated to bringing the perspective of the patient to all aspects of health care.

Glouberman told me a Code Brown story from his point of view. As part of his diagnostic workup, Glouberman was given a CT scan of the abdomen, for which he received an injection of contrast, the dye that radiologists use to spot abnormalities such as tumours. Glouberman says he was informed about the risk of radiation from the scan. He says he was also told in detail about the possible side effects of the dye—with one exception.

"They didn't tell me that I might shit my pants," Glouberman says. "First of all, it's very shocking to suddenly feel that you can't control yourself. You feel horrible and you feel a little bit violated and a little bit ashamed, and you feel a little bit like you are imposing. And after the shit has come out all over everything, they come and clean it up as if it's nothing."

Obviously, the experience was humiliating. Spelling out all of the risks in advance, including the possibility of fecal incontinence, should be Medicine 101. But health professionals might argue that cleaning up incontinence as if it's nothing is our way of trying to be kind to patients like Glouberman by not making a big deal out of it. Talking about it would call attention to it, which might double patients' feelings of humiliation.

On the other hand, we need to appreciate just how mortifying the loss of bowel control is to a patient. This control is a fundamental characteristic of personal autonomy. Losing it is nothing to laugh at.

Another man who has learned to see things from the patient's point of view is colorectal surgeon Marc Burnstein. He says he wasn't always that way: "I hope I wasn't cavalier when I was younger." What does Burnstein think of Code Brown stories today? "Any laughing is, hopefully, going on at a considerable distance from the poor patient who generated it, because they have embarrassment," he says. "It may have been part of a painful experience." He says many of these patients "are older, frailer and sometimes not entirely with it. It's a very sad situation."

Code Brown is no longer amusing to Burnstein for another reason: seldom, if ever, is it self-inflicted. Over the years, I've seen lots of patients induce vomiting. I've seen the occasional patient defecate in the corner of the ER waiting room as a deliberate tactic to gain attention. But I have never seen a patient pretend to have fecal incontinence. I'm not prepared to say it never happens, but I can't find it anywhere in the medical literature.

The patient with fecal incontinence doesn't ask for it any more than the patient with cerebral palsy asks for garbled speech. Laughing at either should no longer be welcome in the culture of modern medicine.

///////

There's overcoming one's disgust at dealing with feces. Then there's getting past one's discomfort with dealing with the part of the body from which feces emerge. Sooner or later, all physicians have to learn how to do a rectal examination. The slang term used by many urologists (who are checking the prostate for enlargement and for a nodule suggestive of prostate cancer) is the *finger wave*. Burstein has done thousands of rectal examinations during his career. He still remembers the first one because of what his teacher did to arrange the opportunity.

"I have to say I don't think it would pass muster today as a way of introducing it to a medical student," Burnstein says. "But in 1977, when I was a medical student, I was at a clinic with a couple of other students and a surgeon. We were assessing a young man whose complaint was a hernia."

An inguinal hernia (sometimes called a rupture) is a noticeable lump in the groin caused by protrusion of the wall of the abdominal cavity with or without a part of the intestine poking through the inguinal canal. Although a rectal is considered an important part of the physical examination, it was probably not that essential in the case of the young man. Nevertheless, Burnstein recalls, every student in his group did a rectal on him.

"I thought having several digital rectal examinations done on a young patient for our education, taught by the fellow who is about to fix your hernia, is not really a free-will, informed-consent situation," says Burnstein.

The notion of a patient being subjected to repeat rectal examinations by students is not new. It even has a piece of slang to describe it: BOHICA, which is short for "bend over, here it comes again." According to Wikipedia, BOHICA is a military acronym that came into regular use during the Vietnam War. Commonly understood as a reference to being sodomized, it apparently signified that "an adverse situation is about to repeat itself, and that acquiescence is the wisest course of action."

It's not surprising that this piece of military argot found its way into the world of medicine. A surgeon who doesn't want his name mentioned and who works in private practice in the Pacific Northwest told me that when he was at the U.S. Veterans Administration (VA), "the veterans who attended the urology clinic would often be guinea pigs for learning residents. BOHICA was the phrase for the prostate clinic. If a patient had a big prostate, the surgeon would be like, 'Come over and feel this.' You would often get one patient who would get three or four or five rectal examinations by different people. The veterans were joking about it. They would say, 'I'm here for my BOHICA clinic.' Like it was funny because they came up with it themselves."

The surgeon says that both the practice of multiple examinations and the nickname continue to this day. He says he has friends who are urologists who describe where residents do general urology training as "the resident BOHICA clinic."

That is as cringeworthy as it is puerile.

///////

The three most offensive bodily fluids health professionals have to deal with are feces, vomit and pus. Of the three, I'd say I'm sickened the most not by the sight but by the smell of pus oozing from an abscess.

"Pus is much worse than poop," agrees Marc Burstein. "It's stinkier and it doesn't wash off as easily."

Burnstein says the worst abscesses he has to drain are known as ischiorectal abscesses, which originate just inside the anus and spread to the buttock. "God bless us, in North America we have lots of big buttocks," says Burnstein. "And you can collect a large amount of pus. Personally, I have not thrown up, but I have had to step out for a minute or two and take a bit of fresh air before I come back in the room. I have seen others whose eyes watered at the odour that you can encounter in these situations."

Nicole Donaldson, the licensed practical nurse has learned not to be fazed by the appearance or the smell of any particular bodily fluid. For eight years, Donaldson worked as a nurse at the Vancouver Island Regional Correctional Centre in Victoria. The people who work there still call it the Wilkinson Road Jail. When she worked at the jail, Donaldson recalls, she was asked by her supervisor to see an inmate who had been transferred to the facility.

"This fella had a pair of shorts on, with very hairy legs. Here I am, trying to pull out stitches. I pulled one stitch and then another. When I pulled the third one, a little pus came out and I was all excited. And he says, 'Oh, wait. Let me show you pus, nurse.'

"He put his left hand underneath his thigh and his right hand on the inner thigh, and he pushed. Pus came out of orifices I didn't even know were there. Pus came out of every stitch. I probably had like a cup of pus with one push. The jail guards knew he was going septic, so they got him to us. We discharged him straight to the hospital for intravenous antibiotics."

For paramedic Morgan Jones Phillips, it isn't pus but vomit that makes him hurl. Beyond *hurling* and *puking*, it's difficult to find medical slang for vomiting alone. There are bits of slang for vomiting in combination with diarrhea. In the United Kingdom, DNV stands for "diarrhea and vomiting" and OBE for "open both ends." Phillips doesn't have slang for a patient vomiting in the back of an ambulance. But he does have an epic story.

"We loaded [the patient] onto the stretcher and were taking him to the hospital," Phillips recalls. A veteran paramedic, Phillips was riding with the patient in the back of the ambulance. He positioned the man on his side so that he wouldn't choke on his own vomit. Protecting the stretcher and the floor of the ambulance from the man's vomit was another challenge altogether. "I was standing up and I had my back to him. Normally, when someone's vomiting, you hear it coming."

When that happens, Phillips is as proficient at reaching for a barf bag and placing it in front of a patient's mouth as Wyatt Earp was with a gun in the Old West. This time, Phillip's patient was unconscious. That meant he didn't make a gagging sound or give any indication of what was about to happen.

"I looked down and he was vomiting," says Phillips. "And I'm right beside him, and it's splashing and it's on my legs. I've never seen vomiting like this. He's already got a big pile on the floor. I put the bag under his mouth, and he fills up the bag, which I have never had happen before. The bag is full, and so I throw the bag into the garbage. I don't have a second bag. I usually carry two, so I must have used one on a previous call and forgot to put a second one in my pocket. So I have to climb over him to get to the shelf to get another bag."

Meanwhile, the patient continued to throw up onto the floor of the ambulance.

"It was probably a good eight inches high and sort of spread like a pyramid and it smelled awful. I was afraid that I was going to throw up. I started to retch."

Phillips got his partner, who was at the wheel, to flick on the lights and sirens—paramedics call them cherries—and get to the hospital as quickly as possible. His partner drove as fast as he would have had there been a child choking to death in the back of the ambulance. Unfortunately, he drove so fast that the neat pile of vomit began to spread all over the ambulance floor.

"As we got to the hospital, we went up this big ramp and then he slammed the brakes on," Phillips recalls. "This tsunami of puke came flying across the back of the ambulance. I jumped onto the bench like a seven-year-old girl seeing a mouse. We ended up being out of service for hours after that because the vomit was everywhere. It was on the walls, it was on the floor. It took forever to clean it up."

With a story like that, it's a wonder anyone would want to become a paramedic.

///////

There is a condition of the lower intestines that attracts its share of stories. Unlike with Code Brown, there is little restraint on the story-telling—and even less empathy for its victims.

We label the condition with the odd euphemism *social injuries of the rectum*. An American colorectal surgeon, Dr. Norman Sohn, first coined the term in an article published in the *American Journal of Surgery* in 1977. The article reported eleven patients with injuries of the rectum and sigmoid colon that were caused by the insertion of a clenched fist—a practice known to men who have sex with men as fisting. Six of the patients in the study sustained cuts to the rectum and four had perforations that required repair in the operating room. One suffered a torn anal sphincter and ended up with incontinence.

Social injuries of the rectum is a lovely bit of medical argot because it can be spoken anywhere. The words are innocuous; only those in the know grasp their true meaning. "I love that expression and I wish I could take credit for it," says Marcus Burnstein, who, like Sohn, trained in colorectal surgery at the Lahey Clinic in Burlington, Massachusetts.

The usual reason people put something through the anus into the rectum is autoeroticism—using the anus and the rectum as organs of sexual gratification. "It's usually somebody doing these things on their own," says Burnstein. "Although we have had patients come in where it was part of a group sex-and-drugs event and somebody did something to somebody else that they would not have done to themselves. These tend to be difficult injuries to treat."

Inevitably, the conversation among health practitioners turns to what objects have been inserted by the social injuries enthusiast.

"Every now and then we'll have somebody come into the ER who has inserted a golf ball or roll-on [deodorant] or zucchini," says Burnstein.

"I've certainly removed lots of strange objects," says Dr. Sid Schwab, a retired general surgeon and author of *Cutting Remarks: Insights and Recollections of a Surgeon.* The book is about his training in the 1970s in San Francisco, where he saw scores of patients with social injuries.

"I had a guy that had inserted a candle," recalls Schwab. "It was at least a foot long and maybe three inches in diameter and it was this hard wax. I just couldn't get purchase on it because anything you tried to grab it with you'd have to spread the jaws so wide that when you tried to close them, it would just sort of slip away. It was so long that, feeling it through the abdomen, it was actually up above his ribs. So I couldn't really push down on it."

Unable to retrieve the candle despite several tries, Schwab got so desperate he began to entertain suggestions. "We just had a parade of people coming in with their ideas on how to grasp it—orthopedic clamps, trying to pass catheters above it and blow the balloon up and pull it back. Nothing worked."

Finally, Schwab did what he was trying to avoid from the outset: he took the man to surgery and removed the object under general anesthetic. "I had to make a little incision in his belly and then I could reach in with my fingers and sort of stabilize it and push it downward and then grab it and pull it out."

There is a certain degree of competitiveness between surgeons as to who has the most elaborate story of what was inserted and how it was removed.

"My own worst experience was a man who came into the emergency department with a large billiard ball in the rectum," recalls Dr. Marcus Burnstein. "A billiard ball is very hard to grasp. We sedated him and couldn't get it out in the emergency department, so we had to take him up to the operating room and give him a general anesthetic to relax the pelvic floor muscles and the sphincter."

Two assistants tried to remove the billiard ball—one pressing on the abdomen and the other trying grasp the ball from inside the rectum using forceps ordinarily used on pregnant women in labour. Their efforts were to no avail. The ball remained stuck inside the upper portion of the rectum.

"Just as we were starting to bring the ball down, the patient coughed," the surgeon recalls with a shudder. "The forceps, the billiard ball, some blood, some gas, and some stool ended up in my lap. We got the ball out, but it was a messy experience."

That is Burnstein's most vivid experience in a long career, but it's not the worst injury he has seen during his residency and his career as an attending surgeon.

"The most serious damage I've ever seen was from a fluorescent light bulb," he says. "It was a long one, like one of those up on the ceiling. They're very fragile. So, naturally, it broke inside him and ripped his rectum, causing lots of bleeding and perforation."

The surgical labour involved in fixing the patient was daunting. "We had to remove a segment of rectum," he says, "and do a colostomy. He had multiple operations over the ensuing six to twelve months dealing with bits of glass and reversing the colostomy. It was a nightmare."

That was bad enough, but there was more. Most inserted foreign objects pose a risk to the patient only. Not so with a fluorescent bulb. "It was very dangerous for the surgical team. Shards of very sharp glass were in his abdomen near blood vessels and near the ureters. It was a disaster. We had to clean up as much glass as we could."

Burnstein told me his stories with admirable restraint. Still, the surgeon, who admonishes young doctors not to spread stories about Code Browns and especially not to laugh at them, feels far less inclined to do so for self-inflicted injuries of the rectum.

"I wouldn't be as aggravated if OR time wasn't so precious," says Burnstein. "These people need help. I shouldn't be grading who needs help, but when operating rooms are being tied up by the removal of a foreign object in the rectum, it's a little annoying."

Worse still, many of these patients are repeat customers. Burnstein refers these patients to psychiatrists, but that does little to prevent future episodes. "In my experience, psychiatrists are not terribly interested in that particular problem. I guess what I should be saying is less that the psychiatrists aren't helpful than that these patients are very difficult to help."

And when it's time to pick up an instrument to help, like all doctors, Burnstein does not have the right to take a pass. For Burnstein, it's just another day at the office.

CHAPTER FOUR

Status Dramaticus

'm an adrenaline junkie. Like most doctors and nurses who work in the ER, I thrive on the excitement of pulling patients back from the brink of death with seconds to spare. I long for patients who bring bona fide life-and-death drama to the place where I work.

Patients like a 41-year-old woman I'll call Andrea, who arrived by ambulance one night. Two paramedics rushed her through the sliding doors past a startled triage nurse and headed straight for the resuscitation room. Andrea was in such a bad state the medics weren't going to wait for the triage nurse to tell them which room to take her to. I saw a blur of stretcher and paramedics round a sharp corner as they hurried into the resuscitation bay and decided to follow.

"Forty-one-year-old G1P0 three days postpartum vag delivery with a PPH," one of the paramedics shouted as she and her partner transferred Andrea to a gurney. "BP 70 by palpation with a pulse 120 and thready."

Andrea had delivered her first-born child, a daughter, three days earlier. She was doing well following her discharge from hospital. The baby girl had latched onto Andrea's breast and was feeding hungrily every three hours. It was during a feeding about an hour before she arrived in the ER that Andrea suddenly felt queasy and started to sweat. She noticed a warm and cozy feeling around her lower torso. For a moment, Andrea felt as though she were relaxing in a hot tub. Then she looked down—past the baby suckling at her left breast— and noticed that the bedsheets around her hips were sopping with fresh blood.

The blood loss had caused Andrea to go into severe shock. Her BP (blood pressure) of 70 was dangerously low. The pulse of 120 was nature's way of trying to compensate for the low blood pressure by getting the heart to work faster. A thready or weak pulse meant that Andrea's heart was losing the battle. I could see that Andrea was in severe shock; she was hemorrhaging to death from a postpartum bleed.

Unlike the bleeding from a first-trimester miscarriage, post-partum hemorrhages (PPH) can be massive. They are the most common cause of maternal death in the developed world. I estimated that Andrea had lost more than a third of her blood volume. This is one of those situations in emergency medicine in which finding the cause— one or a combination of a fatally weak womb muscle, bits of placenta still inside the womb, or blood that does not clot properly—takes a back seat to the ABCs of resuscitation: airway, breathing and circulation.

"Let's start 100 percent oxygen by non-rebreather," I told the nurses. "Two large-bore IVs—one running normal saline and the other lactated ringers—both wide open. Type and cross for eight units of blood. Let's start an oxytocin drip. Let's give her four tablets of tranexamic acid. And call the OBGYN resident stat."

Oxytocin would get the womb to contract. That might stop the bleeding. Tranexamic acid would help stop the bleeding by getting the blood to clot. "Type and cross" is an essential blood test before giving a transfusion. It determines the patient's blood type and tests it against potential donor blood for compatibility. Without this step, the patient could die of a transfusion reaction. The trouble is, it takes at least forty-five minutes to do a proper type and cross. I reckoned that Andrea wouldn't survive that long without a transfusion. Already in shock, her thin blood was no longer properly nourishing her heart, her brain and her other vital organs. Without quick action, Andrea would go into irreversible shock as her vital organs failed.

"Call the blood bank and tell them we need type-specific blood stat," I told one of the nurses. In a dire emergency, we transfuse blood that has been typed and is appropriate for the patient yet hasn't been cross-matched. Type-specific uncross-matched blood is usually available within five minutes of the request. While there is a risk of a transfusion reaction, the risk is worth the life-saving benefit. When type-specific blood is transfused, a cross-match is performed as the blood is being transfused; that way, the transfusion can be stopped immediately if a potential transfusion reaction is discovered.

As the nurses and I were working to save Andrea, it suddenly occurred to me that five minutes had gone by without my speaking to my patient. She was still pale but more alert. Her brow was furrowed and drenched in sweat. The senior resident in obstetrics and gynecology walked briskly into the room as I brought Andrea up to speed.

"Andrea, you're in shock but we're treating that with blood," I said to her. "The gyne resident is here. She's going to ask you some questions and examine you. She will try to figure out where the bleeding is coming from and stop it. I'll let her fill you in on the details."

That was when Andrea's eyes locked onto mine and her pale hand reached over and grabbed my left arm in a vice grip.

"I'm not going to die, am I?"

"Not on my watch," I told her.

The OBGYN made good on my promise, saving not only Andrea's life but her womb.

The rush you feel when you help save someone like Andrea is much better than sex. The rush I get from making a quick diagnosis and getting a patient on the fast track to a save can fill me for days with pleasant thoughts. I get a little buzz each time I tell the story of someone like Andrea. That's the kind of drama that still makes it possible to get through long night shifts—even after thirty years on duty.

⁄⁄⁄⁄⁄⁄⁄⁄

Unfortunately, there's another kind of drama that fills the ER all too often—not from patients who are dying but from those who are convinced they're dying. They are the polar opposites of the Andreas of the world—irritatingly over-anxious in deportment and underwhelming in illness and injury.

We have a rich, disdainful cornucopia of slang terms for patients like these.

A nurse in her early twenties who works in an inner-city setting in the southern United States and blogs under the pseudonym Hood Nurse says such patients suffer from a condition referred to by the amusing name *status dramaticus*. "It refers to patients who come to the hospital and start falling down on the ground," says Hood Nurse. "They put on a whole show for us."

Status dramaticus is a totally made-up bit of slang inspired by the term *status asthmaticus*, which is a prolonged and severe asthma attack that does not respond to standard treatment. Status asthmaticus is a life-threatening condition that demands immediate attention. I've had to intubate such patients and put them on ventilators.

Dr. Jonathan Davis, an ER physician at a small hospital in Georgia, says both he and nurses he works with have used the slang version. "I think in some ways it sounds medical enough that if you were overheard, it wouldn't sound as if you were implying that the person is crazy. Like a lot of words, for us it's just a way of getting humour out of a situation where we're all frustrated."

Unlike status asthmaticus, status dramaticus is all performance and no life threat whatsoever. Call it 2 percent real symptoms and 98 percent exaggeration. I've long been impressed that patients with illnesses that are genuinely life-threatening do not have to convince health professionals that's the case. They let their symptoms and physical signs speak for themselves.

"The person who is making the most noise is usually the least sick, in my experience," says a triage nurse I've worked with for many years. "It's the quiet ones in the corner that you have to worry about."

By contrast, patients with status dramaticus go to great lengths to convince skeptical doctors and nurses that they are seriously ill and in need of urgent medical attention. They spend a lot of time telling you how sick they are, using verbal tone and inflection to add emotional leverage to their presentation.

Since they believe they have a medical emergency, they head for an ER. And the nexus point between the outside world and the ER is the triage desk, where nurses have the unenviable job of quickly sizing up all comers—from patients with hangnails to those at imminent risk of cardiac arrest. Not surprisingly, triage nurses get very good at recognizing patients who magnify their symptoms. Dr. Erin Sullivan, a veteran ER nurse who spent many a shift at a triage desk before switching careers to become a physician, is currently doing a residency in family medicine in Saskatchewan. She refers to these patients as *dying swans*: "The dying swans are the ones that go into histrionics with the triage nurse in the waiting room."

The Dying Swan, a ballet created in 1905 by Russian chor-eographer Mikhail Fokine, depicts the last moments in the life of a swan. Describing a patient as a dying swan implies utter disbelief at both the magnitude of the patient's symptoms and their import. Sullivan says dying swans often use flourishes such as wearing dark glasses and moaning or yelling about their symptoms. Like their stage namesakes, dying swan patients know how to get a response from the audience. "They know how to play the part," says Sullivan, "clutching themselves, dry heaving into garbage bags and things like that."

The role of the Dying Swan was created for renowned prima ballerina Anna Pavlova. Triage nurses use *dying swan* to refer only to female patients. They have another name for the guys. They're said to have the "XY chromosome." "A man and a woman both come to the ER with kidney stones at the same time," says Sullivan. "They have the same size kidney stones, but you will only hear the man. The man is moaning and rattling the bed frame and yanking the call bell. And the woman is sort of lying there quietly. A nurse will ask what's wrong with the guy and someone will answer, 'He's got the XY chromosome.' And everybody laughs."

That story would get a laugh in most ERs. The gender stereotype of the wussy man crying about his kidney-stone pain is considered acceptable by many health professionals—hardly surprising, given the tendency to treat men with contempt when they fail to suck it up.

What may surprise you is the proclivity of some people on my side of the gurney to extend the same contempt to members of certain ethnic groups. In parts of the United States with a large Hispanic population—now the nation's largest ethnic or racial minority—it isn't uncommon for some doctors and nurses to refer to patients of Hispanic origin who are loudly suffering from pain by the slang term *status Hispanicus.*

The *Urban Dictionary* defines *status Hispanicus* as "when a large Hispanic family gets together at a hospital to support a member of their family with a minor injury and have a sustained freak-out attack to show the support."

Another slang term, *ay-tach* (pronounced "eye-tack"), pokes fun at the way Hispanic patients vocalize when they are in pain. "When they're expressing pain, instead of saying *ow* or *oh*—what English-speakers might say—they say *ay*," a resident explains.

The resident says that Hispanic patients tend to repeat *ay-ay-ay* in staccato fashion over and over again—the inspiration for *ay-tach* (sometimes called *Tachy-ay*). Ay-tach comes from the medical term V-tach, short for ventricular tachycardia, a rapid-fire, life-threatening heart rhythm disturbance.

Dr. Zubin Damania, a hospitalist (a doctor who cares for patients in hospitals) in Las Vegas and a well-known medical satirist who writes, produces and stars in his own videos as ZDoggMD, doesn't use such terms. But he remembers hearing them when he was a resident at Stanford University School of Medicine in California, which is home to a large Hispanic population. "Oh yeah, they exist," says Damania. "It's big among the younger doctors and the residents and interns. It's interesting because your first instinct is to think this is a racist kind of a moniker."

Damania says that ay-tach is "a way of describing a slightly obese, middle-aged Latina who has some non-specific pain—a gall bladder or a functional [pain not caused by a recognized illness] abdominal pain where we don't figure out what it is, or back pain. It also happens with pregnant women in labour."

Dr. Peter Kussin, the Duke University Hospital respirologist, remembers similar terminology when he was a student at Mount Sinai School of Medicine (known today as the Icahn School of Medicine at Mount Sinai) in New York City back in the 1980s. "I can still get away with talking about how at Mount Sinai back then there were rooms of four or eight patients," Kussin recalls. "On the women's rooms, you'd go in and you'd have Tachy-ay in one corner and Brady-ay in the other." *Brady-ay* —based on a bradycardia, or abnormally slow heart rhythm—also is slang for a Hispanic patient moaning the Spanish word *ay* over and over, but at a much slower rate than the patient in Tachy-ay.

"We were pretty liberal in our use of slang—even at the limits of what would be acceptable," says Kussin. "And then it disappeared."

Kussin says that in the late 1980s, state regulators and professional organizations such as the American Association of Medical Colleges recommended that the use of slang be banned from training programs because it lacks professionalism and compassion.

"I don't think it's feasible to speak like that today," says Kussin. "I think you have got to steer clear of race. You have got to steer clear of ethnicity. You have got to steer clear of gender."

Damania says that status Hispanicus has started to disappear but he still hears ay-tach from time to time, mostly from doctors and nurses in the ER.

///////

Doctors tend to like patients who are stoics more than we like those who demonstrate that the pain they feel is making them suffer. Having pain from a bona fide cause cuts no ice with many of my colleagues.

"When we say someone's inflated their symptoms, it's all our personal judgment," says Georgia ER physician Dr. Jonathan Davis. "Of course, pain being a subjective thing, someone stubbing their toe could really feel as bad as someone with a ruptured aorta."

Deep down inside, patients in status dramaticus probably know they aren't dying. It's just that they almost never admit it. They leave that frisson of doubt that maybe—just maybe—they do have a serious medical condition. I keep praying for a miracle of modern medicine that would have patients arrive in the ER with a sign on their foreheads that says something like "Symptom Exaggerator." I'm still waiting.

Like me, Hood Nurse says triage nurses have to be on guard in case the patient with status dramaticus has a serious condition. "I think some people genuinely think something a lot bigger is going on," says the inner-city nurse and blogger. "They're just really freaked out and stressing, but for the most part, I think a lot of times people are just being ridiculous."

Reinforcing the notion that status dramaticus is a performance, such patients raise their game in front of a live, captive audience of fellow patients, family members and bystanders in the waiting room.

"It tends to happen a lot more when the waiting room is full," says Hood Nurse. "They just kind of see the writing on the wall and they want to get through the doors [to a doctor] a little bit faster."

From her perch at the triage desk, Hood Nurse says, she sees patients with status dramaticus all the time. She says one—a young woman in her twenties I'll call Wanda—came into the hospital complaining of abdominal pain. "Once we got her triaged, she was still trying to get up and roll around," says Hood Nurse. "I've got visitors and housekeeping staff coming up to me telling me that this lady won't get off the floor. She just refused to take a seat or co-operate in any way."

Hood Nurse says she did not ignore Wanda. In fact, she left the triage desk to find the doctor on duty to order an injection of a pain reliever to make her more comfortable while she waited. But that didn't satisfy Wanda. "She literally came up to the window in our little triage desk area. She was asking why she had to wait and I was explaining to her that we've got a lot of people here who are very sick and have been waiting a really long time—like eight hours."

Wanda didn't buy that explanation one bit. Frustrated at the ongoing wait, she became agitated. "She was literally having a hissy fit like a three-year-old. It was complete and utter meltdown."

Triage nurses are nothing if not patient. They assess dozens of patients to see who goes in now and who can wait, keep track of those who have to wait hours before getting through the sliding doors, not to mention placate their families. Hood Nurse has seen many patients like Wanda and her abdominal pain—patients who demand to be treated immediately. The nurse says she has been spat upon and been subjected to verbal abuse.

What happened next was a bravura performance that earned Wanda the label *status dramaticus.*

"She just kind of very gently lowered herself to the ground and pretended to pass out," recalls Hood Nurse. "I had to have my charge nurse come out there with ammonia caps [smelling salts] to get her to suddenly be 'revived.'"

That certainly got the waiting room's attention; every eye was glued on Wanda, every person wondering what was going to happen next. To the astonishment of many who watched her fall to the floor, Hood Nurse simply ignored Wanda after she was given the smelling salts. The tactic worked. "She figured out that her antics weren't going to work," says Hood Nurse. "She got up, sat in a corner, spent about an hour texting and then she unplugged her phone and went home."

Hood Nurse is being modest. It takes experience to recognize that a patient like Wanda is in status dramaticus—and it takes guts to fend off bystanders who rush toward the patient to render assistance.

"This whole scenario plays out in front of all these visitors," Hood Nurse recalls. "There was one guy who was really sweet. He thought she must have finally passed out from the pain. He offered to help to get her up off the floor. I had to reassure him that she was going to be okay. He was completely taken aback—just astounded that somebody would do that."

A genuine fainting episode—not the kind Wanda had—is known by the clinical term syncope, a brief loss of awareness from which the patient recovers spontaneously and does not require treatment. Faints range in severity from a benign loss of consciousness called vasovagal syncope to a life-threatening form called cardiac syncope. Patients who experience the latter usually fall face first as they faint, and often break their noses or other bones of the face when they fall. For Hood Nurse, the fact that Wanda protected her face by sliding gingerly to the floor was the tipoff that she was faking it.

And faked fainting is not the only pseudo-serious condition that Hood Nurse has witnessed. She has also seen patients develop a case of something she and her nursing colleagues call spontaneous paralysis.

"Honestly, it's not even that notable anymore because we get one per shift," says Hood Nurse. "They act like they can't walk. Or they'll come in for some complaint that's not related to paralysis and yet they require a wheelchair. They may come in with generalized weakness. Maybe they've been vomiting. They act like they can't move, when there's no physical reason why that should be happening.

"It often happens when they're accompanied by family. They'll act like they're too weak to do anything. They want to go to the bathroom but they refuse to stand up. They make you lift them up on the bedpan."

As with someone who pretends to faint, the hallmark of spontaneous paralysis is how quickly the performance ends. "The doctor will come in and tell them there's nothing wrong with them and tell them they're going home," says the triage nurse. "They literally stand up and walk out of the ER."

Unfortunately for ER physicians and nurses, very few dying swans or patients with status dramaticus or spontaneous paralysis get up and walk out of the waiting room. Most of them make it through the sliding doors.

A lot of anxious patients inhabit the ER. According to the Anxiety and Depression Association, 40 million Americans have an anxiety disorder—nearly one in five Americans aged 18 and older. Patients with an anxiety disorder are three to five times more likely to seek medical attention than people who aren't anxious. All told, they cost the U.S. more than $42 billion a year. Add in stress-related illnesses and lost productivity, and the cost is close to $300 billion a year. The problem of anxiety is also reflected in high rates of consumption of anxiolytics (anti-anxiety meds) such as Lorazepam and Alprazolam.

There's even a bona fide clinical term for what's afflicting people who come to the ER repeatedly in search of reassurance about their health: it's called health anxiety. While most people experience momentary jitters about their health or the health of a loved one, health anxiety is a more pervasive state of fear about disease and dying that becomes so preoccupying that it interferes with the ability to work and enjoy life. According to one report, up to 30 percent of the population experiences intermittent fears about their health; from 3 to 10 percent suffer from significant health anxiety.

The triggers to a bout of health anxiety include everyday symptoms such as a skipped heartbeat, a headache, a wave of nausea or a bout of abdominal pain. Like many ERs, the one in which I work has an area called the rapid assessment zone, or RAZ. The laudable idea behind the RAZ is to identify patients that we can assess, treat and send home without requiring a referral to a specialist or a stay in hospital. On the plus side, the RAZ concept has significantly improved our ability to see a large segment of the patients we see in very timely fashion.

Another thing I've noticed is that triage nurses have an uncanny ability to put many of the patients with health anxiety into RAZ—prompting one of my colleagues to say that RAZ really stands for "rapid anxiety zone." Not a shift goes by without seeing a patient or two in the RAZ with health anxiety. The trouble is, these patients don't come in complaining of health anxiety. They come in complaining of chest pain, shortness of breath, dizziness, heart palpitations, abdominal pain and sometimes nausea. The main clue to the true origin of their maladies is the fact that they are young and otherwise healthy. That rather vague observation is not much to go on.

The other clue is how patients with health anxiety react to expressions of skepticism about the seriousness of their symptoms. If I had a dollar for every time a patient has said "I only come to the ER if it's serious," I'd be very wealthy. Patients with health anxiety are often repeat customers (a subset of what we call frequent flyers). When the ER physician tries to get such a patient to reflect upon his or her many visits, the patient often replies, "But this is the first time I've come in with *this* problem."

I find that patients with health anxiety get offended when you call them on it. They are very skilled at playing the ultimate trump card: that they may be right about having a life-threatening illness. If I'm meeting them for the first time, I have no idea whether they are truly ill or indulging in a pattern of behaviour. So, like most colleagues I know, I take them at their word and order tests such as CT scans of the head, chest and abdomen that I wouldn't dream of ordering if I knew the patient was merely anxious.

In a supreme irony, many such patients undergo CT scans—utterly oblivious that doing so increases the risk of cancer caused by the radiation needed to do the scan. A 2013 study published in *JAMA Internal Medicine* found that most patients undergoing CT scans underestimated the amount of radiation delivered during a scan. A third of those surveyed who were getting a CT scan didn't even know the test exposed their body to radiation. Just one in twenty believed the scan would increase their chance of getting cancer.

A 2007 study by researchers from the National Cancer Institute estimated that the 72 million CT scans done in the U.S. that year would result in 29,000 future cancers. And yet, of those surveyed in the 2013 study, most were more concerned about when they could eat following the test and whether their hospital parking costs would be reimbursed.

On the other hand, for many of the worried well who inhabit the RAZ , the dosage of radiation from a CT scan is perfectly fitting: it's one more thing to get anxious about.

///////

There's a subset of anxious patients that deserves special mention. Unlike the status dramaticus patients who seem to pluck free-floating anxiety out of thin air, the patients I'm talking about have a bona fide medical condition; it's just that they're more anxious about it than others.

Here's a made-up encounter with a patient that represents a scenario that I've seen so many times in my career I can't even count them. A patient I'll call Iris comes to the ER with shortness of breath. Iris has asthma, a frequent cause of difficulty breathing. Over the course of my ER career, I've probably seen about 2,500 patients with asthma. I've read as many articles and attended as many continuing-education lectures on asthma as almost any other condition. I've read the current guidelines and I'm quite comfortable treating patients with asthma.

But Iris is different. For one thing, Iris is pregnant. Asthma is no more prevalent in pregnant women than in the general population. Like all patients with asthma, pregnant women with the condition can develop respiratory failure and can even die of it. The bottom line—whether the patient is pregnant or not—is that you have to treat an asthma attack.

When I examine Iris, I can hear loud wheezes emanating from her chest. She is breathing at a brisk thirty breaths a minute. My immediate concern is that, without treatment, she'll soon get tired of working so hard to breathe and go into respiratory failure.

The treatment of severe asthma in pregnancy is virtually identical to that of non-pregnant patients. We prescribe inhaled beta adrenergic bronchodilators such as Salbutamol, which open up the air passages, along with inhaled and oral corticosteroids such as Prednisone to reduce the inflammation in the airways that is part and parcel of an asthma attack.

Unfortunately Iris is paralyzed with anxiety about taking *any* medication for asthma because she is pregnant. She doubts my word at every turn.

"I don't want to harm the baby," says Iris.

"If you can't breathe, that will harm the baby too."

"What are you proposing?"

"I'd like to start you on inhaled bronchodilators as well as steroids," I reply.

"Are steroids safe in pregnancy?" she asks.

"Yes, they are. We give them to pregnant women all the time."

"But Prednisone has a Level C risk," says Iris. The look in her eyes and the tone in her voice say that from now on she'll take everything I say with a grain of salt.

Let's back up a bit. The U.S. Food and Drug Administration puts prescription drugs for pregnant women into one of six categories according to the risk of harm to the baby. Category A drugs have not demonstrated any risk to the baby based on "adequate and well-controlled studies." Category B contains drugs for which no risk has been found in studies in animals but for which there are no adequate and well-controlled studies in humans. Category C drugs have shown an adverse effect on the fetus in animal studies but there are no adequate and well-controlled studies in humans. According to the FDA, the potential benefits of Category C drugs "may warrant their use in pregnant women despite potential risks."

Category D contains drugs for which there is evidence of human fetal risk, "but potential benefits may warrant use of the drug in pregnant women despite potential risks." Category X, the final category, is the FDA designation for drugs with evident risks of harm to the fetus that "clearly outweigh potential benefits."

Prednisone has not been formally assigned to an FDA risk category. However, a byproduct of Prednisone called Prednisolone has been given a Category C designation because of conflicting evidence of harm from some animal studies. I consider this a technicality. In my many years of ER medicine, I have never withheld Prednisone from pregnant women who needed it, and have never seen a colleague—including experts in asthma—do so either.

What Iris hasn't told me is that she knows that Prednisone is a Category C drug because she has looked it up online. Dr. Google has struck again!

I am a big believer in patients using the Internet to get engaged in their own disease management. It makes me uncomfortable when patients ask a question to which they already know the answer because they looked it up. Iris has set up the doctor-patient relationship on a patently false test of her own making. It's the test that demonstrated to me that Iris was not only pregnant and had asthma but she had health anxiety to boot.

The other thing about health anxiety is that for doctors it often leads to decision paralysis. A pregnant woman comes to the ER with pains in her chest that get worse when she takes a deep breath. The pain could be due to a strained back muscle or a bruised rib. It's probably one of those inexplicable pains that arrive and depart mysteriously.

Unfortunately though, pregnant women also happen to be at increased of having a pulmonary embolus (PE) or blood clot on their lungs—a potentially fatal condition. In the absence of any other proven cause, I'm often forced to rule out a PE by ordering a CT scan of the woman's chest. A CT scan is often the most accurate and safest way to rule out a clot. And that's where the trouble begins.

I can't begin to calculate how many hours I've spent in the ER trying to reassure pregnant women that a CT scan of the chest is unlikely to cause cancer in their unborn child—to little or no avail. So they sit in their cubicle—afraid to go home lest they have a blood clot and afraid to have a CT. So powerful is their sense of helplessness born of anxiety that I've some patients ruminate on this decision for hours.

When it comes to anxious patients, I must admit that I have a bit of a character weakness. I tend to get defensive when questioned closely by overly worried patients. I'd be very surprised if I'm the only one who finds hyper-anxious patients very challenging.

To the calm patient, Dr. Google is a source of helpful information that promotes constructive engagement with health professionals. To those with health anxiety, it's an enabler and a magnifier of fear and doubt.

I'm hardly the only health professional who feels that way. Hood Nurse says she and her colleagues often see the kind of patients they have nicknamed Dr. Google and Dr. WebMD. "Usually, we're the second opinion," says Hood Nurse. "But we're not valued."

She recalls a woman coming into the ER "who had all the classic symptoms of a sexually transmitted disease. She had decided (based on Googling her symptoms) that she had cervical cancer." Hood Nurse says she tried to reassure the woman that it was unlikely she had cancer. "In some cases, people are relieved when they hear that," she says. "But in a lot of cases, they just think that we nurses are idiots because they know better, or their smartphone knows better."

She recalls hearing the father of a girl brought to the ER with a diabetic emergency argue with the doctor about the dose of insulin. She says he came armed with knowledge obtained from the Internet. "This is somebody who had absolutely zero medical training," Hood Nurse recalls. "The stuff that the father was suggesting we do probably would have killed her."

Hood Nurse says that in her experience, patients with health anxiety are more likely to try out their Dr. Google skills on nurses than on doctors. That leaves it up to ER physicians to convince the patient that Dr. Google has the wrong diagnosis or the wrong treatment.

"If the doctor is interested in convincing them, they can convince them," she says. "People kind of dismiss a lot of the things that the younger nurses say, particularly if they're female. The majority of our doctors are male. Sometimes if people hear it from a male, somehow that has more credibility. I don't think they recognize that, but they somehow hear it with more authority and they're okay."

⁄⁄⁄⁄⁄⁄

According to a Canadian Psychological Association fact sheet, some people are born predisposed to health anxiety. High family stress during childhood can lead to inordinate fears about health and illness. Some kids learn to be anxious by following their parents' example. The illness and death of a close relative during childhood can make a person grow up to have a health anxiety.

The problem of health anxiety is also being played out against skyrocketing levels of other anxiety disorders. Why North America is so anxious these days is a matter of considerable debate. Taylor Clark, author of the 2011 book *Nerve: Poise Under Pressure, Serenity Under Stress, and the Brave New Science of Fear and Cool,* says it's not the precarious economic recovery following the 2008 recession or an uncertain job market. In a blog post in 2011, Clark cites three factors that make a lot of sense to me.

The first is what Clark calls the Bowling Alone effect, named after *Bowling Alone: The Collapse and Revival of American Community,* by author and political scientist Robert D. Putnam. Clark says North Americans tend to move far away from family and lose a steady source of emotional support that helps alleviate anxiety: "Another factor that adds to this problem—especially among young people—is our growing reliance on texting and social media for community, which many psychologists say is no substitute for real human interaction."

The second factor Clark cites is information overload. Clark says the public is exposed to many more bits of news than ever before—more than some neuroscientists believe the human brain can absorb. And much of that information, says Clark, is alarmist in nature—especially health scares, which range from emerging infections to cancer risks attributed to cellphones and wi-fi networks.

The third reason, Clark says, is an unhealthy habit of dealing with negative feelings such as nervousness and sadness by fighting to ward them off instead of just letting ourselves experience them.

That last one tracks with what I see almost every shift I work in the ER. Instead of acknowledging that they fear being sick, I see patients who fight to ward off the fear by looking to the physician to magically take the fear of illness away. To the doctor, that usually means doing a diagnostic test that rules out a worst-case scenario. But indulging patients by searching for the worst-case diagnosis reinforces their conviction that they were right to worry in the first place.

The unhealthy way of dealing with fear is to become helpless in the face of it. In medicine, we call it "failure to cope." The slang term is *dyscopia*—a witty play on legitimate medical terminology. The prefix *dys-* means "bad, painful or disordered." Dyspnea means difficulty breathing. Dysphagia means difficulty swallowing. And *dyscopia* is an invented term that means difficulty coping.

Dr. Erin Sullivan, the former nurse and budding resident in family medicine, uses the term *hypocopenemia*—a nonsensical bit of slang that means low level of coping skills in the bloodstream—to mean the same thing. "You might look at their medical presentations as not that severe, but they are just not handling the fact that that they are in the hospital," says Sullivan.

Sullivan's explanation reminded me that sometimes the term *dyscopia* is used to refer to patients who can't cope with a battery of blood tests and other invasive procedures. Often, the term is reserved for a family member who has been the patient's caregiver and is finding the job increasingly challenging.

A triage nurse told me that one night a young woman brought in her mother, who had chronic heart failure. The woman announced to the nurse that she was leaving her mother at the hospital because she could no longer look after her. She said she could no longer perform daily nursing tasks like weighing her mother every day to make certain she wasn't retaining water—a sign of worsening heart failure. The nurse also remembers how the daughter reacted when told her mother was not going to be admitted.

"She just got so angry with me, as if I personally was making the decision," the nurse recalls. "I just had to keep explaining to her that this is just not the way our system works."

The other reason for dyscopia is anxiety. If you think anxious ER patients drive us crazy, try the anxious parents of infants and young children. A couple of veteran pediatric ER physicians who didn't want their names used (and who are mothers themselves) schooled me on that.

"We talk about hypoparenting," says the first physician, whom I'll call Sally. "We talk about acopia or hypocopia when there's a psychosocial element to the presentation of the child, when a parent could be doing a little bit better for their kid."

If dyscopia refers to bad or difficulty coping, the prefix a–, as in acopia, means the complete absence of coping skill. The term sounds technical enough that it can easily be said within earshot of parents without attracting their attention.

How does Sally know that parents are inadequate after just meeting them?

"That's a very provocative question," says Sally. "Sometimes we think it's true if we see recurrent visits for a similar problem without plans having been made and no follow-through. From our perspective, when it's two in the morning and you're telling the parent the same thing for the tenth time, it's hard sometimes to be sympathetic or empathetic."

Wendy, the other pediatric ER physician, paints this picture of a parent who suffers from acopia: "I go to see a child with a fever. I ask mom how long the fever has been going on and she says for less than an hour! The child hasn't had any antipyretics [drugs that reduce fever] at home. Just like that, she has demonstrated to me the inability to do any problem-solving before coming to the ER."

What impact does that have on doctors like Wendy?

"Well, after the twentieth fever in a row where they're telling me the same spiel over and over again, I start to lose a bit of empathy."

But Wendy's her greatest fear is an unspoken one: that after twenty children in a row with fever, she might lose the diagnostic edge that enables her to detect the one child with a life-threatening infection.

"I guess we feel confident that 95 percent of fevers in small children who are immunized and look well are viral. We are confident in our history and physical examination. When the kid's running around the department, he usually doesn't have meningitis. Pediatrics is very gestalt-driven. As soon as they walk in the door, you have a pretty good sense of whether the kid's sick or not."

I certainly hope so!

///////

As I've said, I have trouble dealing with anxious patients. So too does the culture of medicine, which mounts an almost immunological reaction to the anxiety with which patients leverage their illnesses. I've given a good deal of thought to what it is about anxious patients that people who practise medicine find so toxic. For one thing, anxiety is insatiable. After all, it is frequently based on a hypothetical worst-case scenario of illness that is often disproven only in retrospect. Doctors and nurses find it difficult to get in synch with anxious patients. We meet them in the here and now, while they exist in the worried future of scary diagnostic possibilities or the regretful past of prudent health choices not taken.

But the most important reason physicians can't stand anxious patients is what anxiety does to the medical mind. Anxious patients make health professionals feel anxious too. There is growing evidence that the brain activity of health-care providers can mirror that of their patients.

In a 2013 study published in the journal *Molecular Psychiatry*, researchers at Harvard University did an intriguing experiment in which eighteen doctors were exposed to pain from a heat source while their brains were being monitored using functional magnetic resonance imaging (fMRI). When the physicians experienced relief from the pain, a portion of the brain known as the ventrolateral prefrontal cortex lit up.

In the second part of the experiment, the doctors, again hooked up to fMRI machines, became observers while a researcher posing as a patient was exposed to the same heat-source pain that the physicians had experienced. The doctors were tricked into believing they were either relieving the patient's pain or permitting the patient to suffer.

The results were telling. When they believed that the patient was experiencing pain, there was no change to the physicians' fMRI scans. But when they believed the patient was experiencing pain relief, the very same ventrolateral prefrontal cortex that had lit up when the physicians got pain relief lit up again when the physicians believed that the patient was getting pain relief.

This experiment demonstrated that under the right circumstances, the brain activity of doctors mirrors that of their patients. If that is true of physicians whose patients experience pain relief, it's probably also true of physicians whose patients are anxious.

Anxiety makes the doctor less likely to consider all of the pertinent diagnostic possibilities and consequently more likely to make mistakes that harm and even kill patients.

In some instances, the impact over-anxious patients have on the medical staff can be so profound that doctors and nurses are tempted to use drugs to medicate the anxiety away. When ER patients are agitated, it's considered medically appropriate to give them intravenous medications to sedate them. On the other hand, it would probably be considered malpractice to give an anxiolytic drug such as Lorazepam to patients simply because their anxiety is making it more difficult for the doctor to think!

That may be true in the ER, but in the operating room, it's a different ballgame, says Dr. Jay Ross, an anesthesiologist. "An anxiolytic like Midazolam can often take a really anxious patient down a few notches," says Ross. "They're nice and calm and relaxed or just quiet."

Not surprisingly, patients about to undergo surgery are very anxious. When that happens, they hold their breath, making it difficult for the anesthesiologist to prepare the patient to be intubated and placed on a ventilator. It's medically appropriate to give patients a medication that helps them relax enough to breathe deeply before intubation. But there's another side to the use of sedating drugs in the OR that's in more of a grey area. Although most patients undergoing surgery receive a general anesthetic, some receive a spinal or epidural anesthetic instead. Spinal and epidural anesthetics work by numbing the part of the body where the operation takes place; the two techniques are different, but both involve delivering medication through a needle inserted in the lower back.

These forms of anesthesia have fewer side effects. Patients usually recover faster and go home from hospital sooner than those who receive a general anesthetic. But they aren't ideal when the patient is having extensive surgery.

Of course, the other difference compared with general anesthesia is that with spinal and epidural anesthesia, the patient is wide awake. And talking. Sometimes, far too much for the surgeon and the anesthesiologist to tolerate.

"The patient is just wondering if everything is okay," says Ross. "Or they're just chatting about the news or whatever happens to be on their mind. But sometimes, they're excessively chatty to the point where they're actually distracting you from doing your job.

"They try to look over the drapes if that's possible, or start to move their legs around. They're getting tired of lying in a particular position. Their arms are moving. They're trying to scratch their nose. It's getting a little dangerous for their own safety because you don't want them to disrupt the surgeon, who may cut something accidentally. So we try to keep things safe."

Ross says one piece of coded language used in the OR is a signal that tips off the anesthesiologist that the patient is becoming a distraction and needs to be given a drug to quiet him down. The code phrase is SFU 50, which sounds scientific. But like a lot of medical slang, the root of it is a neat pun, says Ross. The phrase, which Ross says he's heard but doesn't use, is inspired by the scientific term ED 50 or Effective Dose 50, which is the drug dose that produces the effects for which it is administered in 50 percent of patients. "In anesthesia," says Ross, "there's the SFU 50 dose. That is the dose [of sedative or anxiety-reducing medication] at which 50 percent of the patients will shut the fuck up [or SFU]."

Until Ross mentioned it, it would never have even occurred to me to administer sedating drugs just to get an awake and anxious but non-agitated patient to keep quiet! I polled some of my ER colleagues, and they said pretty much the same thing.

///////

A 2013 article in *Psychology Today* lists treatments that patients can use to deal with health anxiety. These include confronting one's fears and learning to face worries about illness realistically. My favourite is to not seek absolute certainty or safety.

Useful though these suggestions are, they won't work in a busy ER where people like me don't have the time to get to know patients who might be more anxious than ill—or who might not.

The truth is, no matter how seductive it might seem, I dare not snuff out the anxiety of my ER patients. Every once in a while, their fear of imminent death is bang on.

One night many years ago, I was working in a community hospital when a 60-year-old woman I'll call Abigail came to the ER complaining of sharp pain in her chest. An electrocardiogram and a blood test showed no evidence of a heart attack.

"Good news," I said to Abigail. "Your tests are normal. You can go home now."

Instead of being relieved, my patient looked and sounded worried.

"Please don't send me home," Abigail begged in a quiet voice. Her brow was furrowed and her tone and manner told me she meant it.

It was a busy afternoon in the department. I had a lot of patients to wrap up before I could go home. Now Abigail was adding to my list of unfinished business.

I sighed and began to retake the history of her symptoms. The first thing I thought of was to rule out pulmonary embolus, a blood clot on the lungs. I ordered a lung scan—a standard test at the time to look for a pulmonary embolus.

Late that evening the lung scan was completed. The result of the scan was what we call indeterminate; it failed to show a blood clot and yet the scan was not completely normal. I told Abigail she could go home, and this time she did so without protest. That night, she died in her sleep. An autopsy showed that Abigail had an aortic dissection—a tear in her aorta that caused her to have pain.

If I had diagnosed Abigail's dissection, she could have been saved. Instead, she was sent home. There, her weakened aorta broke wide open and she bled to death in seconds.

Abigail's plea not to be sent home sounded like the importuning of a woman in status dramaticus. Instead, it turned out to be—literally and figuratively—a *cri de coeur* that will haunt me for the rest of my life. She reminds me that when it comes to patients in status dramaticus, SFU 50 is one thing I dare not use, tempting though it may be.

CHAPTER FIVE

Failure to Die

In the novel *The House of God,* the most famous offering of medical slang by far is the word GOMER. Author and slangmeister Dr. Stephen Bergman defined GOMER as a patient who is frequently admitted to hospital with "complicated but uninspiring and incurable conditions." The definition is bland, but the acronym immediately and irrevocably touched a raw nerve with residents, attending physicians, nurses and other health-care professionals for several reasons.

GOMERs are usually old, demented and sick with half a dozen or more illnesses pressed into a package of decrepitude. For good measure, throw a pinch of utter futility into the mix. Doctors can perform all manner of medical miracles on a GOMER, but what you end up with is a GOMER who is less ill than before, but a GOMER nonetheless.

Oh, and one more thing: unlike young people in the prime of life with serious illnesses, GOMERs don't die (at least they don't die easily). So true is that statement that Bergman made "GOMERs Don't Die" top of the list of the Thirteen Laws of his fictional hospital.

Make no mistake. If you're a health professional, unless you love geriatric patients, chances are you can't stand GOMERs. And that's a huge problem in health care today.

By the year 2030, according to the U.S. Administration on Aging, 19 percent of Americans will be 65 and older. Currently, the Alzheimer's Association estimates that five million Americans have Alzheimer's disease; by 2050, the number is expected to rise to 16 million. They may be your grandparent, your mother or father, a favourite uncle or aunt, or even you or your partner.

The loved one you see as special is a patient seen by most health professionals as someone who takes up a valuable bed on a packed hospital ward. And increasingly, they ask: "Why are you here?"

And "Why haven't you died?"

///////

11:35 p.m. The Bunker.

"We've been consulted from emerg to see a 93-year-old man with aspiration pneumonia," a senior medical student I'll call Cynthia reported to the senior resident. "Am I going to get a history out of him?" asked Cynthia, who was on call for general internal medicine.

"Why don't you go see for yourself," said the senior resident with a chuckle.

It's the job of the on-call team of budding internists to assess, diagnose and, if necessary, admit patients who arrive at the emergency department.

"I went to visit the patient. He was in end-stage dementia," Cynthia remembers. "He was blind in both eyes, completely bedbound and non-verbal."

The senior med student quickly sized up that her patient did have aspiration pneumonia, a disorder in which the lungs have become inflamed due to the presence of oral and stomach contents. There are many causes—strokes, multiple sclerosis and intoxication, to name three. But by far the most common cause is advanced dementia associated with old age. That was the first thing to come to Cynthia's mind as she pondered her new assignment.

The old man's complexion was blue. He was breathing rapidly in a physiologically instinctive way to make up for the lack of oxygen passing through the alveoli, the tiny membranes deep inside his lungs. He was also gasping for breath. With each sharp intake of air, the man made a thick, wet, gurgly sound that meant his airways were filled with mucus and pus. His heart was galloping along in a vain effort to make up for the lack of oxygen by sending deoxygenated blood coursing through his arteries ever faster. Without quick treatment, Cynthia's patient was on a path to almost certain death from suffocation.

Her assessment finished, the medical student went back to the Bunker to confer with her teammates. As she presented the cold, clinical facts, a simple choice emerged: Give the man antibiotics and delay his death or hold back the antibiotics and make the man comfortable.

"This is cruel, to keep this guy alive," Cynthia argued to her teammates inside the Bunker. "I don't want to step him up to a more potent antibiotic. I think that this guy should return home [to die]."

There were murmurs of support, as Cynthia and the team spoke in a cold and spare way about the futility of keeping the man alive. What strikes her later as she recalls the episode is that they were *joking* about the choice; to the team, the fact that there was a choice at all was amusing. The idea that there was any point to the man being saved was *that* preposterous.

Deliberations complete, Cynthia stepped outside to discuss the man's prognosis with his family, and to ask what they thought he would want were he able to speak for himself. What she remembers most about the encounter with the family is that she had to shrug off the amusement she'd just shared with her teammates and present the "options" in a deadly serious tone of voice—when the team had decided there was only one appropriate option: no treatment.

The family chose the antibiotics, and the man lived.

"You try and persuade people to do what you think is appropriate," she concludes about her conversation with the family. "I think there's a real disconnect between what goes on back there [in the Bunker] and then how we portray ourselves out there. I don't think patients are at all aware of that."

What also bothers me about the case Cynthia described is that these life-and-death discussions took place around the man, as if he didn't exist. To the team, in a cognitive sense the man had already died. The man was too demented to realize it himself.

Cynthia's patient was old and decrepit. He had dementia, and no amount of medical care could change that. What the team in the Bunker thought he needed was some TLC at home or in a nursing home and die. Instead, he got good acute-care medicine—powerful antibiotics, advanced airway management, and lots and lots of blood work—all of it, from their point of view, irredeemably futile.

That's what it means to treat a GOMER.

///////

The origins and derivations of GOMER help shape the meaning in the culture of modern medicine. The word can actually be found in the *Merriam-Webster Dictionary*, defined as "medical slang, usually disparaging: a chronic problem patient who does not respond to treatment." Stephen Bergman says GOMER was already in use when he was an intern back in 1973. That same year, in an article titled "The Language of Nursing," published in the journal *American Speech*, the American author and English professor Philip C. Kolin offered this mention of GOMER in the lexicon of medical slang: "Those patients who require long-term care and who are usually sent to a nursing home are known to the RN as gomers."

The July 1972 issue of *National Lampoon* referred to GOMER as "a senile, messy, or highly unpleasant patient." According to John Algeo's book *Fifty Years Among the New Words: A Dictionary of Neologisms 1941–1991*, GOMER might go back as far as the 1950s.

The derivation of GOMER is somewhat unclear. In *The House of God*, GOMER is an acronym for "get out of my emergency room." But Algeo's *Dictionary of Neologisms* says that on the West Coast, GOMER stands for "grand old man of the emergency room."

In his 1982 book *What's the Good Word?*, William Safire quotes Dr. Adam Naaman, a physician in Clifton Springs, New York, who says GOMER derives from the Hebrew verb *l'gmor* which means "to finish." Safire quotes Naaman as saying a GOMER is a patient "in the process of finishing his existence on the face of this earth." Naaman says that the word "started in New York City, where many Jewish house-staff officers [interns and residents] sprinkled the medical language with words from Hebrew and Yiddish. Obviously, WASP interns had to find other explanations for the term, and hence the acronym was invented for 'get out of my emergency room.'"

In "The Language of Nursing," Philip C. Kolin speculates that GOMER possibly derives from *gomeral*, a Scottish word meaning simpleton or fool. In a 2006 blog post, Michael D.C. Drout, the Prentice Professor of English at Wheaton College in Norton, Massachusetts, declared he was "as close to certain…that the actual etymology of 'Gomer' in medical slang is not an acronym, but from the character 'Gomer Pyle.'"

The title character of the television show *Gomer Pyle, U.S.M.C.*, which ran on CBS from 1964 until 1969, was an unsophisticated yet kindly gas station attendant who joined the Marines. The character was first introduced on *The Andy Griffith Show*. The simple-minded Gomer Pyle served as a foil to a by-the-book drill instructor named Sgt. Vince Carter.

Drout wrote that in the early 1970s, GOMER was medical slang for a stroke patient, head-trauma victim, or someone afflicted by senile dementia. On his blog, Drout says he's pretty certain of the origin of GOMER because his father was an intern and resident at New York Hospital from 1973 to 1976—the same time that slangmeister Stephen Bergman did his internship. Drout says his parents often entertained his dad's colleagues, who told stories about the hospital.

"Although I heard the word 'Gomer' used very often, I never heard the 'get out of my emergency room' acronym and, if it had been invented, I am sure I would have heard it: med students, interns and residents loved that kind of thing," Drout wrote on his blog.

The point is that GOMER means different things to different doctors. If you're a patient's family member, it might be worthwhile trying to figure out which of the definitions I just gave you is meant by your loved one's doctors. It might just give you an important clue about where they're coming from.

Though just about every doctor and nurse knows the word GOMER, the term is rarely if ever used now. That's because it has made its way into the public vernacular. GOMER has been used on TV shows including *Scrubs* and *ER*. When that happens, it's no longer insider slang, so it gets discarded.

Today, health professionals use a multitude of other slang terms instead. Dr. Zubin Damania has honoured the word GOMER by inventing a variation. "We call that *status gomaticus*," says Damania, echoing *status dramaticus*. "It basically means that this guy is never going to get well enough to resume any quality of life but he's never going to die."

There's a multitude of newer slang terms for GOMERs—each of which illustrates something about these patients that doctors find very frustrating. At the top of the list is the reality that once GOMERs are admitted to hospital, it can be difficult—bordering on impossible—to get them out. Not surprisingly, they're called bed blockers.

Bed blocker is the slang term for a patient admitted to an acute care hospital for acute medical problems—issues such as dehydration and infection. The acute problems are treated, and the patient is designated for transfer to a rehabilitation hospital to receive additional care before returning home. Or the patient may be earmarked for transfer to a long-term care facility for the rest of her life. Either way, the patient must remain in the acute care hospital until an appropriate bed opens up elsewhere. As long as these patients remain in hospital, they block another patient from being admitted.

When a bed is blocked, an internist can't admit new patients and surgeons can't admit patients who need operations. That hurts doctors in their wallets.

The impact of bed blockers on the overall functioning of the health-care system can be enormous. In Canada, a 2011 report by the Wait Time Alliance found that bed blockers take up one in six hospital beds—causing ERs to fill up with acutely ill patients and resulting in the cancellation of elective surgeries. The report found that, on average, one bed blocker admitted to the ER denies access to patients seated in the waiting room at a rate of four per hour.

"Bed blocking generates problems throughout the health-care system, from longer wait times in the ER to poorer health outcomes for patients from accelerated functional decline, social isolation, and loss of independence," wrote Dr. Jeremy Petch, an expert in biomedical ethics and health policy at the Li Ka Shing Knowledge Institute at Toronto's St. Michael's Hospital, in a 2012 blog entry at healthydebate.ca.

According to wisegeek.net, *bed blocker* is primarily British, Australian and Canadian slang. The circumstances and the reasons may be somewhat different, but bed blocking is a growing concern in the United States as well. Bed blockers cost hospitals as much as $1,500 per patient per day. The added financial burden threatens the already shaky financial viability of publicly funded hospitals in the U.S.

Given the stress on the system that these patients cause, physicians' antipathy toward them begins to make sense. Take it as an article of faith that internists are the hospital physicians most likely to have bed blockers on their wards. Still, it's a term that disturbs budding geriatrician Dr. Nathan Stall. "These patients are not in hospital because they want to be there, and they're not trying to cause a problem to the system," says Stall. "I think, really, the system is failing them."

In Canada, the "fix" for bed blockers is to designate them for placement in a nursing home by reclassifying them as Alternative Level of Care, or ALC. It's a way of shuffling the patient off a team's list of acute care patients. The term reminds me of what Fortune 500 companies do when they write off bad loans and delinquent creditors. ALC has become the new name for GOMER. In the Bunker, the designation is cause for celebration. "Often, there's definitely high-fiving when someone is made ALC," says Nathan Stall. "That's an accomplishment. They're pretty much off your list."

Once that happens, the patients no longer receive active treatment and blood testing. They may not even have their vital signs monitored. Stall knows of instances in which the care of such patients is so neglectful that they suffer serious complications. "The team kind of pops their head in once a week. I know that geriatricians have said that these patients have been horribly mismanaged—things that people have not picked up on."

Something like that could be happening to a loved one of yours who resides in that limbo state between acute patient and nursing-home resident.

"I've seen things where something more aggressive could've been done but more so the typical geriatric preventive measures could've been done," says another resident, who didn't want her name used. She recalls a patient who was admitted to hospital by an internal medicine team. The patient was bedridden and spent his days lying flat in bed. "His wife was feeding him while he was lying down, which put him at great risk for aspirating his meal."

The patient stopped breathing; he had to be placed on a ventilator and ended up being transferred to the ICU, where he died. What bothers the resident is that the death could have been prevented by having the patient sit up during meals. "I have this horrible feeling that maybe one simple thing could have saved his life," she recalls.

///////

From the foregoing, you might be tempted to think bed blockers don't exist in the U.S., a view that is depressingly untrue. In some places, including New York, Texas, Florida and California, there's a growing list of bed blockers that are next to impossible to remove from hospital wards to nursing homes.

In January 2012, the *New York Times* reported that hundreds of patients have "languished for months and even years" (that's right, years) in New York City hospitals, despite the fact that they are considered by doctors to be well enough to be discharged or at the very least discharged to a nursing home. The reason? The patients are illegal immigrants.

Under New York state law, if patients don't have a lawful address, public hospitals aren't permitted to discharge them to shelters or to the street. And while Medicaid pays for emergency care for illegal immigrants, it does not pay for long-term care. The result is that such patients—like their ALC brethren—remain in limbo in acute care hospitals for years. One such patient in New York has remained in a hospital on Roosevelt Island for a staggering thirteen years, according to the aforementioned *New York Times* article.

Bed blocker is a polite term for such a patient. At one of the top hospitals in America, they called them rocks. "A rock is a patient that cannot move because they're just stuck," says a resident in internal medicine who agreed to speak to me only if I withheld his name. "If we have a lot of rocks, we call it a rock garden," he adds.

An attending physician in the ICU at the same hospital told me that rocks are not uncommon at the hospital because farms in the region hire a lot of illegal immigrants who arrive with no money and no family to care for them.

The attending ICU doctor recalls a case from early in her career that taught her a lesson about the dangers of uprooting rocks. The patient—an illegal immigrant from Mexico—had a bad accident and was admitted on a ventilator to the ICU. Eventually, he recovered enough to be transferred to a long-term care facility. As was the case with other such patients, the man had no insurance.

"We have trouble getting our regular patients on ventilators, who have insurance, into a facility," says the attending doctor, whose identity I'm protecting because of what happened.

Having no place in the U.S. to send the patient, the hospital arranged to transfer him on a ventilator—which he depended on to be able to breathe—to a hospital in his native Mexico. They got the man's family members to come to the hospital to accompany him on the journey home.

"We got the patient back to Mexico on the ventilator," she recalls. "And when he got there, the hospital immediately disconnected him from the machine," she says. As a result, the man died of asphyxiation.

In the U.S., we might call what was done at the hospital in Mexico manslaughter, if not premeditated murder. It was a hard lesson for the doctor who told me the story.

"It was real eye-opener for us because we had spent all this time and energy getting it arranged," she says. "We don't do that anymore."

Instead, they let slang terms like *rock* and *rock garden* express the frustration they feel about these all-but-immovable patients.

////////

Doubling the frustration about the patients they can't remove from hospital beds, doctors are also frustrated that they had to admit them in the first place. There is a strong thread among residents and attending physicians that GOMERs just aren't worthy of their knowledge, their skill and their time. They label such patients as suffering from "failure to cope."

Often used to describe over-anxious patients, *failure to cope* is also used to describe GOMERs who are not particularly ill and (if younger and more able bodied) could almost certainly be sent home. But age and infirmity have made the patients unable to master a new diet or a new regime of medications, or to attend follow-up appointments.

"They're not eating and drinking as well as they should and not looking after their personal hygiene," says Dr. Nooreen Popat, until recently a resident in internal medicine at McMaster University in Hamilton, Ontario. "So they need to come into hospital and be looked after by some allied health-care personnel, or perhaps have the social worker get involved."

Some residents don't have the luxury of calling on a social worker. Instead, they have to perform many of a social worker's functions, which makes many bristle.

"I feel like *failure to cope* is a very derogatory term in that it is blaming the patient for some sort of failure," says Dr. Amanda Gardhouse, a resident in internal medicine at McMaster and one of very few young physicians committed to becoming a geriatrician. "Our system is not designed to deal with all the multiple medical issues that geriatric patients bring to the table. We're not really sure what's going on, so we're going to call this failure to cope. It's very sad."

Andrew Burke, who trained in internal medicine at McMaster, refers to failure to cope by two other slang terms. "Well, that would be a 'social admission,'" says Burke. "Someone with a 'positive suitcase sign.'"

Just about every doctor and nurse has heard if not used *positive suitcase sign*—sometimes called the *positive Samsonite sign* in reference to the manufacturer of luggage. The phrase takes a clinical trope—*positive* in medicine means the presence of an abnormal finding (for example, "the urine dipstick test was *positive* for blood") and combines it with *suitcase* to create a slang term that means the patient made an unscheduled trip to the ER but had time to think about packing a suitcase.

"In the emergency department, a 'positive suitcase sign' literally means when you go in to see a patient, you see their suitcase on the floor," says Dr. Rick Mann, a family physician. "The patient or the patient's family have already determined that the patient will be coming into hospital—regardless of what their diagnosis is or whether there is or is not a medical problem."

The reaction among emergency physicians and nurses to the patient with a positive suitcase sign ranges from amusement to profound irritation.

"One of the frustrations is that there isn't necessarily one clear thing that we can do to solve failure to cope," says Dr. Clarissa Burke.

"You know it isn't just a matter of fix your knee pain now, you'll be able to walk around and do everything. They still wouldn't be able to look after themselves."

Another reason the positive suitcase sign bothers physicians so much is that it's perceived as a demand to be admitted to hospital—and as a direct challenge to the doctor's authority to decide. The patient or family member who insists that the patient be admitted may become known as demanding—but patients will not be admitted on demand.

If you're thinking of bringing a suitcase to the ER, best to leave it in the car.

///////

Frustration about having to care for patients doctors think don't require their knowledge and skill animates much of medical slang. But even recognizing *that* requires some insight on the part of physicians. All too often, they search the patient for small medical problems such as a bladder infection or a slight drop in hemoglobin or sodium levels. These problems sound serious; in reality, they're trivial because they don't harm the patient. Fixing them won't make the patient better, but will earn the doctor some money and a sense of accomplishment.

There's a nickname for such behaviour, says medical resident and future geriatrician Nathan Stall. Call it "kicking the can down the road." To a team of residents, kicking the can down the road means fixing little things yet doing nothing substantive to address the reasons a patient was admitted to hospital. "We kind of tidy them up," says Stall. "We say they have an acute kidney injury, so we give them intravenous fluids. We put them on antibiotics for pneumonia. We hear a heart murmur and so we order an echocardiogram.

"But their main problem might be this complex functional psychosocial thing and we're just in such a rush, and too overburdened to do it, that we don't actually get to the problem that's causing these people to come to the hospital."

Stall says he sees residents and attending physicians play kick the can down the road almost every day. An example that sticks in Stall's mind is of an old woman who had fallen and broken her pelvis. She was confused and delirious. "Her admitting doctors heard a heart murmur and ordered an echocardiogram," says Stall. "They were rehydrating her with intravenous fluids. They were testing her urine to see if an infection was the reason why she was delirious."

All of these actions made it seem as if the doctors were taking good care of the patient. Stall says they completely missed the underlying issues that made the woman fall and break her pelvis in the first place. As Stall dug deeper, he learned that the patient had gone downhill during the past year following the death of her beloved pet, a cat who was the woman's main source of companionship.

"The woman was depressed, so she stopped going for walks," says Stall. "That made her less in shape and more likely to fall. To sit down and actually figure out what was wrong with her was not actually that challenging, but the difference that it could make on her life is huge."

I've heard doctors say they don't have the time to delve into the factors that make an old man depressed. I would suggest that the real reason isn't lack of time so much as a lack of interest in fixing the problems that bring frail seniors to hospital in growing numbers.

Kicking the can down the road epitomizes the search by doctors for medical diagnoses that either don't exist or aren't worth fixing. Sometimes, doctors try to fix things that either can't or shouldn't be fixed. The slang term used to describe that is *flogging*.

Dr. Zubin Damania says he first heard of flogging in connection with patients who are war veterans. The Veterans Administration (VA) operates the largest integrated health-care system in the United States. It has more than 1,700 hospitals, clinics, community living centres and other facilities. Damania cut his medical teeth looking after veterans from the Second World War and more recent conflicts.

"They had every single chronic disease in the world," says Damania. "They had PTSD [post-traumatic stress disorder] and all the other stuff that goes with it and they all were smokers. So they were super-enriched with pulmonary disease and end-stage congestive heart failure. As veterans, they didn't ever want to give up. Their families never wanted to give up. So we just flogged somebody with treatments. It was totally counterproductive, but it would keep them alive."

The word *flogging* has been likewise adopted by residents and attending doctors in internal medicine in reference to GOMERs. Duke University Hospital pulmonologist Dr. Peter Kussin says he first heard it during his own residency in New York City. "One of my teachers in pulmonary would put it in his notes and on his admission orders," Kussin remembers. "We knew exactly what he meant."

As Kussin recalls, flogging had a humorous yet therapeutic meaning—to give a patient with asthma several different kinds of drugs to try to relieve his shortness of breath, as in pulling out all the stops.

There's treating a patient aggressively to try to stave off death. Then again, there's treating a patient *unto* death. Even that concept has its own slang term: *cheech*. According to the online *Urban Dictionary*, *cheech* is "ordering every radiologic and lab test imaginable to diagnose a confounding (or at some institutions, not-so-confounding) illness. In noun form (also known as cheech-bomb), it refers to the panoply of tests itself."

Damania says he heard *cheech* and *flog* a lot when he went to med school at the University of California at San Francisco. "It means every single medical intervention is going to be done to this guy until he cries uncle or the family says, 'No, no, no more,'" says Damania. "The cheech was often done to GOMERs, but it didn't have to be. We often flogged a GOMER or flogged somebody who wasn't a GOMER. It all kind of swirled in the same yucky mess of doing things *to* people instead of *for* them."

An attending ICU doctor at one of America's top hospitals told me the famed medical facility has been known to cheech patients. As one of the major health facilities in the southern United States, the hospital frequently gets referrals from smaller, rural hospitals to transfer patients who are beyond hope. "We accept these patients knowing there's nothing we can do to save them," she told me.

And when that happens, the doctors at the leading hospital feel they need to justify accepting the patient by performing all manner of invasive tests—even redoing ones that were done quite competently by the referring hospital. Keep in mind that by definition, these patients are already sick and near death.

I think the doctors would do better to have a realistic chat with the family about the patient's prognosis.

⁂

Of all the modern synonyms for GOMER, the most pointed one goes right to the heart of the matter.

"You've probably heard the term *failure to die*, haven't you?" Dr. Donovan Gray asked me rhetorically. Gray, a veteran ER physician in Winnipeg, Manitoba, with more than twenty years of experience, is author of the book *Dude, Where's My Stethoscope?*, a collection of short stories about his career and his view of modern medicine.

Failure to die (FTD) is a play on the bona fide medical phrase "failure to thrive," which refers to an infant—and sometimes a frail elderly patient—who is unable to maintain an ideal body weight. Gray says he has heard it used many times by general internists and emergency physicians. "The mind is long gone, but the body is chugging along," he says. "Maybe [the patient] gets pneumonia or something." The table is set for a fairly quick and painless death—except nobody told the patient.

"They just keep on going for weeks and weeks or months," says Gray. "You're just thinking that it would be so much kinder for this person to pass away. It's a bit grim but it is accurate."

FTD is not the only phrase that captures the sense among doctors and nurses that such patients are simply putting in time until they expire. At some hospitals, these patients are called walkers—the term used on the popular TV series *The Walking Dead* to refer to zombies. *Walker* is a bit of irony, as the vast majority of walkers are bedridden.

In *The House of God*, Dr. Stephen Bergman introduced slang to describe patients at or near the end of life. "O Sign" refers to a patient so far gone that her mouth remains open in the shape of the letter *O*. A variant of the O Sign is the Q Sign, in which a patient's tongue protrudes from the side of the mouth, forming the letter *Q*. Both slang terms are still used widely by doctors and nurses.

Kris Schultz, an oncology nurse with more than a decade of experience in Massachusetts and, more recently, in Georgia, recalls a colleague filling her in on a patient. "She kind of shrugged and said that he's starting to exhibit the Q Sign. She turns to me and does the face. I remember giggling hysterically—so much so that I had to quiet down because there were patient rooms right outside of the nurses' station and I didn't want anybody to think I was laughing at the idea that somebody was dying."

Note that Schultz wasn't concerned that she enjoyed the mimicry, only that bystanders might observe her laughter.

Failure to die implies that the patient's continued existence is utterly futile. Medical futility is a very hot topic in hospital corridors these days. Faced with an aging population and ballooning health-care costs, more and more doctors wonder whether they can continue to take on all comers in need of life-saving treatment.

The concept behind medical futility is a simple one: no treatment will put things right with the patient. The problem is that there are no universally accepted criteria for futility in the corridors of medicine. That's the maddening part of this discussion. When it comes to cracking the genetic code of a disease or coming up with ultra-precise clinical criteria for giving a stroke patient clot-busting drugs, physicians are models of exactitude. But when it comes to medical futility, doctors and nurses can only say they know it when they see it. All too often, medical futility is a judgment made by a health professional based on what he or she—not the patient—would want.

"For me, I think, 'Oh, my God, I would not want to live like that,'" says Gray. "I tell my children about once a year to pull the plug on me if I get to that sort of state. They have no illusions about that. But that's me, not everyone. Some people view life as sacred even if it's not meaningful anymore. And some people say even though their grandpa's completely demented, if they put a spoon of Jell-O in his mouth, he eats it. So that means that he has some satisfaction in life, and so we'd like to keep going with all possible treatments."

I have a personal stake in what Gray is talking about. My mother has advanced Alzheimer's disease. For many years, she has been unable to speak and unable to tell us her wishes. My late father, my sister and I were forced to guess on a number of occasions. For the past three years, she has been unable to feed herself, and so the three of us, plus a growing list of hired caregivers, took turns feeding her. On some level, we *supposed* she got some pleasure from the taste of food on her tongue. A while back, my mother was admitted to hospital with dehydration. The internist on call gently chided us for calling an ambulance instead of letting her die. "Perhaps you should consider not doing that next time," he said.

As a family, we have decided not to "keep going with all possible treatments," as Gray put it.

I've never been convinced that front-line doctors and nurses care all that much about medical futility per se. After all, futility doesn't come out of their pocketbooks. Publicly funded health care, private, or a mixture of the two—it doesn't matter. Futile or not, we get paid to care for patients with dementia.

Put that way, FTD and futility are in the same ballpark as cheeching and flogging in that all of them mean serving up treatments when you know they won't bring the patient back. The only difference is that cheeching is initiated by doctors; it's called futility when it's requested by patients or their families.

Either way, it's not good for the person who is often forgotten: the patient.

///////

The slang we doctors use to describe older patients is an expression of frustration with everything from what's wrong with them to their very existence. But it doesn't explain *why* we're so frustrated.

One obvious reason is that we mirror the ageism in society at large. In the past few years alone, researchers have documented that ageism affects the treatments seniors receive in heart disease, diabetes and cancer care, to name just three conditions. Sadly, much of the blame goes to the fact that medical students receive little education in gerontology and spend little time with good role models.

This may shock you, but today's doctors are astonishingly ignorant about how to take care of older patients. We don't know what we're doing. And when that happens, we get frustrated.

Ignorance would be forgivable if we resolved to do something about it. But that's not the case. A 2012 report by the Rand Corporation documented a critical shortage of geriatricians in the U.S.

The trouble is, very few young doctors want to become geriatricians.

"I was told that I was wasting my talents, that I was too smart to be doing something like that. And how could I pick a specialty where I wasn't actually helping people?" Nathan Stall, who has chosen geriatrics, told me.

Instead of smart and enlightened care, the growing numbers of seniors get a dollop of disdain laced with slang.

CHAPTER SIX

Swallowers

I f you have pneumonia, I can put you on the antibiotic azithromycin
and you'll be feeling better in three or four days. If you come into
the ER with a near-lethal level of potassium in your bloodstream,
I can order up a cocktail of treatments to bring the level down fast.
Show up with a pneumothorax—an expanding pocket of air between
the inside of your chest wall and your lung—and I can puncture your
chest wall with a tube or a pigtail catheter, evacuate the air pocket and
you'll be breathing better in three or four minutes.

But if you come to the ER with schizoaffective disorder, psychotic break or borderline personality disorder, I—and most of my
colleagues—could talk to you for three or four years and not have a
clue as to what makes you tick, let alone how to help you. But that
doesn't mean we don't practise medicine on emotionally afflicted
patients. Far from it.

A patient I'll call Rhonda (a composite of many such patients)
has been coming to various ERs for years. She's been diagnosed
with severe borderline personality disorder (BPD), a chronic, largely
incurable psychiatric condition marked by extreme depth and variety
of moods, unstable interpersonal relationships and a fragile sense of
self. People with BPD—mostly women—go through periods in their

lives when they try to harm themselves. The most severely affected may commit suicide.

Rhonda is one of the most practised swallowers I have ever met. To call her the Super Elite of frequent flyers, patients who visit the hospital over and over again, is to trivialize her accomplishment. Think of her as if she'd joined the fictitious American Airlines 10 Million Mile Club—as actor George Clooney did in the 2009 film *Up in the Air*. Rhonda swallows pins of all kinds, kitchen knives, spoons, forks, house keys and the occasional USB flash drive.

Once or twice a year, Rhonda visits an ER to have the large number of objects she's swallowed removed. It's become a ritual that is as mindless for the doctors and nurses who look after her as it apparently is for her. As soon as she arrives, the doctor on duty orders an X-ray of Rhonda's abdomen to locate the things she's swallowed. Then the gastroenterologist is called to insert a gastroscope and remove the offending bits. It's done under a light general anesthetic, often administered by an ER physician like me.

I have spent as much as an hour or longer administering vast quantities of the anesthetic drug propofol to keep patients like Rhonda sedated long enough for the GI fellow to snare the various objects.

Professional sword swallowers are probably the only people in the world with any useful insight into this bizarre practice. In 2006, Brian Witcombe and Dan Meyer did a survey of sword swallowers that was published in the venerable *British Medical Journal*. According to their survey of some fifty English-speaking sword swallowers, most spent hours a day for months, even years, perfecting their craft. The swallowers said they learned to suppress the gag reflex by repeatedly putting fingers down their throats. They then learned to swallow spoons, paint brushes, knitting needles and plastic tubes before progressing to bent wire coat hangers. Then, it was on to swords.

When a pro or determined amateur swallows a sharp object, the principal danger is that it will pierce or perforate the esophagus or stomach. Mortality from perforation can be as high as 30 percent, but few accidental deaths of professional sword swallowers are reported.

When patients like Rhonda come to the ER, most of the time the GI specialist is able to fish out the objects they have swallowed and we send them home. Although such patients have a psychiatric disorder, rarely if ever do we ask a psychiatrist to see them. Rhonda's personality disorder is so intractable to therapy that a consultation with a psychiatrist is generally considered pointless. The cumulative cost in health-care dollars of this recurring exercise would probably run close to $1 million, virtually all of it paid for by publicly funded health care.

As harsh as this may seem, few doctors and nurses would shed a tear if the Rhondas of the world perforated a vital organ and died as a result. The sense I get from ER personnel is that anyone who would do what Rhonda does, and waste ER time and facilities in the process, merits contempt. Even her name is irrelevant. Instead, we use slang to reduce what she does to herself to a stereotype. She isn't Rhonda; she's a swallower.

Rhonda's a subtype of a much larger group of patients who frequent the health-care system and baffle us endlessly. Doctors and nurses label them *psych patients*.

One guy who has picked up on the lingo is Jason Quinn, a first-year resident in psychiatry who at one point wanted to be an ER physician like me. "'Psych patient' is code for annoying, a bother, a time sink and somebody who's not going to get better and is damaged and wasting the space in my emergency department or on my floor," says Quinn.

Quinn recalls enjoying his rotation in emergency medicine and especially the excitement of being the first person to lay eyes on a patient. But, unlike ER physicians who recoil at psych patients, Quinn was drawn to them—the sicker the better. He remembers one ER physician whom Quinn regarded as an otherwise excellent teacher who confronted Quinn about his interest in patients with mental health problems.

"Why do you want to see the psych patients?" Quinn recalls the ER physician asking him. "They're not going to get better. Why don't you just let one of the senior residents deal with them and then psychiatry will see them?"

Quinn was disturbed by the way the ER physician dismissed not just the patients but Quinn's interest in them: "To me, that said something about the attitudes that are held throughout the rest of medicine about psychiatry and psychiatric patients."

Turns out the attitude Quinn encountered from his ER mentor—along with some very pejorative language—has been prevalent in the halls of medicine for a long, long time.

///////

Pejorative terms for the mentally ill have existed in non-medical literature for centuries. *Mad as a March hare* dates back to Chaucer's *The Friar's Tale*, most likely written in the 1380s, and in Shakespeare's *King Lear*, written about 1605, Edgar disguises himself as the beggar known as Mad Tom. More than 250 years later came one of the most popular references to madness, in Lewis Carroll's *Alice's Adventures in Wonderland*, published in 1865. Lost in a forest, Alice asks the Cheshire Cat for guidance. Many of you will remember his famous advice: "'In *that* direction,' the Cat said, waving its right paw, 'lives a Hatter: and in *that* direction,' waving the other paw, 'lives a March Hare. Visit either you like: they're both mad.'"

As mentioned earlier, in his 1973 catalogue of nursing slang, Philip C. Kolin wrote that nurses called patients with manic depression (now called bipolar affective disorder) "manics" and those with schizophrenia "schizzes," and they described patients agitated by psychiatric disorders as "bouncing off the walls." Modern medicine is rife with such psychiatric slang. Not surprisingly, many of the terms are invented and used by health professionals who do not specialize in psychiatry.

As a veteran psychiatric emergency nurse, Sarah Reynolds has been observing her ER colleagues for years. "We all have slang, and I think it's especially prevalent in the emergency room just because of the turnover," says Reynolds. She admires the ability of ER nurses and doctors to see and treat a wide variety of patients—urgent and otherwise. But toss an agitated and unpredictable psychiatric patient into the mix, and medical staff seem to have a particularly hard time.

"Psychiatric patients are seen to be overdoing it and taking up an awful lot of time," she says. "If patients are disruptive, intoxicated or manic, they take time and resources. They often frighten people. They have to be restrained. They're a burden on the resources and frighten the other patients."

And make no mistake: psychiatric patients *are* disruptive—especially the ones having a psychotic episode.

An ER nurse told me about a psychotic patient who was hearing impaired. "We wrote out our questions to him. He read them and then answered in this very loud voice. He wanted me to help him make a phone call to his friend. I dialled the friend and gave the phone to him. He told his friend that a spirit had made it necessary for him to enter the hospital."

Suddenly, the patient screamed that he was in grave danger. "He's bellowing this, and I'm looking around, and all of these little old ladies are looking at him." The patient had to be restrained.

Reynolds says it's hardly surprising patients like that generate some colourful ER slang. "Crazy is used often," says Reynolds. "Or bat-shit crazy. Nuts is used very often. So are wing nut, wacko and psycho."

Dr. Grumpy, a pseudonym for a neurologist who blogs about his experiences, says he uses similar slang. "You occasionally see the phrase JPN for 'just plain nuts,'" he says. "I think I've used that one here and there. It's usually in conversations with other doctors at the hospital."

Like *swallower*, such slang words indicate that some health professionals find psychiatric patients mysterious, unfathomable and more than a little frightening. Reynolds has tried to get inside the heads of those who use them—beginning with *crazy*, which is used in different ways.

"It can mean anything from 'I think this patient is anxious and might require a chat' to 'Shut this person up. They're driving me nuts and they're upsetting everybody else,'" says Reynolds. "I think sometimes it is unkind and it diminishes the patients' needs and treats them as a nuisance."

I suspect the label says more about the health-care provider than it does about the patient. Like the triage nurse, when I say a patient is crazy, I mean that the patient is making *me* crazy.

Interestingly, Reynolds says her psychiatric colleagues use *crazy* as a form of code to indicate to the ER staff it would be better if mental health professionals took over. But as first responders, my ER colleagues and I usually end up having to manage patients in the throes of a psychotic break without immediate assistance from experts in psychiatry. When that happens, the patients are not only a danger to themselves but to ER personnel and bystanders. If we can't calm such patients by soothing them with words, we sedate them with injections of drugs such as haloperidol and Lorazepam.

"We call the drugs 'vitamins,'" says one veteran ER physician. "There's vitamin L for Lorazepam and vitamin H for Haldol."

These drugs most assuredly are not vitamins. Turning a treatment into slang by calling it a vitamin is a favourite trope of ER physicians. I think it detaches us emotionally from what we're doing to agitated patients in severe emotional distress. Like a vitamin, it makes us feel more powerful.

As Sarah Reynolds suggests, despite their outward bravado, ER personnel harbour deep insecurity about dealing with agitated patients. We don't feel particularly competent in assessing and treating them. The slang calms us, just as the sedating drugs calm our patients.

///////

The world of psychiatry has its myriad diagnoses, labels and slang. Often, it can be difficult to know where one ends and the other begins. The bona fide diagnoses come largely from one source, the *Diagnostic and Statistical Manual of Mental Disorders* (*DSM*). Often described as psychiatry's bible, in terms of the Secret Language of Doctors it might also be described as its thesaurus. The volume is meant as a tool to help psychiatrists diagnose patients, providing them with definitions and criteria patients must meet before they can officially be labelled with such illnesses as depression, psychosis or autism spectrum disorder.

The American Psychiatric Association (APA) published the first edition of the *DSM* in 1952. It listed 106 mental disorders. The *DSM* was born in part out of a need for a common language; practitioners across the country needed to understand each other. "There was great confusion and variability in diagnoses of mental disorders because diagnostic systems were about as varied as the institutions

and individuals that created them," wrote James Sanders, author of
A Distinct Language and a Historic Pendulum, an article about the
evolution of the *DSM*.

The creation of the *DSM* was also an attempt to order an
unorderly division of medicine. "To be sure, psychiatrists were aware
of their inability to demonstrate meaningful relationships between
casual elements and the presence of particular behavioral signs or
symptoms," wrote Gerald Grob, author of the article *DSM-I: A Study
in Appearance and Reality*. "Yet social and cultural roles of medicine
required that all physicians—psychiatrists and others—provide some
explanation of disease processes."

It's more than fifty years later and scientific explanations for
psychiatric illness remain elusive, and that leads to a well-entrenched
dichotomy in the world of medicine.

"There's already this ingrained idea that psychiatrists are dealing
with non-organic problems," says Jason Quinn, the first-year psychiatry resident. "Not real things. Not real medicine."

The words *organic* and *non-organic* have legitimate meaning
in the world of medicine. However, doctors most often use them as
pieces of medical slang.

What Quinn calls "real medicine" refers to treating diseases
found in living tissue as opposed to the mind. Think conditions
such as diabetes and kidney failure, organic problems for which
a definite pathophysiology exists in patients' bodies. Non-organic
medicine, on the other hand, implies that the disease is not a part
of patients' bodies but is in their minds. It is often used as slang for
psychiatry.

Part of the problem is that, unlike cardiology or orthopedic surgery, psychiatry is a relatively new field of study. It's got some catching up to do, says Robert Klitzman, a psychiatrist and bioethicist at
Columbia University Medical Center in New York City. Klitzman is

the author of several books, including *A House of Dreams and Glass: Becoming a Psychiatrist* and *When Doctors Become Patients.*

"It's much harder to study autism, schizophrenia, depression, bipolar affective disorder and anxiety disorder than kidney or bone disorders," says Klitzman. "We don't know as much about how these disorders work on a physiological level. The science is moving along rapidly but is not as advanced as other areas in which it's easier to intervene."

It's the absence of hard science that makes it easier to denigrate the field of psychiatry.

"When we say 'non-organic,' we immediately delegitimatize that disease as a real thing," Quinn says. "And it becomes very stigmatizing because even the language of medicine says it's a non-organic disease and therefore not a real disease."

Other terms are also used to distinguish psychiatric from non-psychiatric patients. *Structural* illnesses exist in the body; *functional* illnesses exist in the mind. Both words have bona fide meaning in the world of medicine. But more often than not, the word *functional* is slang that implies a patient's symptoms are imaginary.

Another slang term used to label patients, especially by non-psychiatrists, is *supratentorial.* Like a lot of slang, it is a bona fide word. The *Merriam-Webster Dictionary* defines it as "relating to, occurring in, affecting, or being in the tissues overlying the tentorium cerebelli." So supratentorial refers to medical problems occurring in and around the brain tissue, such as strokes and brain tumours.

Used as slang, supratentorial means the patients' symptoms are all in their minds. A veteran ER physician who practises in western Canada told me she learned the word from an attending internist who was teaching her and some fellow students at the bedside of a patient who complained of dizziness. "The internist said right in front of the patient that her symptoms were supratentorial," she recalls.

My ER colleague says the internist used the term to denigrate the patient's symptoms. "The internist was trying to tell us that the patient was not going to be a good teaching case," she says. "The sense I got was that we were going to listen politely to her story and then move on to the next patient."

Even more telling is the fact that the whole psychiatric versus non-psychiatric split is an artificial construct. Psychiatric diseases—from schizophrenia to Tourette's syndrome—have an organic basis. It's seldom "either/or" but rather "both."

"You can scan the brains of people suffering from depression with functional MRIs that show change in various brain circuits," says Quinn. "You can see clearly how it is, in fact, an organic pathology."

Still, many health-care workers think psychiatric patients don't have real diseases. So what does that say about those who choose this branch of medicine?

"I don't feel like our field is as prestigious as primary care," says Jason Lai, a psychiatric nurse who works at a mental health agency in Ohio. "I feel like primary care [family and internal medicine] probably thinks of us as not as scientific as them. And in some ways it's true, because medicine understands the brain the least."

The fact that much of psychiatry isn't rooted in science makes many doctors, including psychiatrists, uncomfortable, and contributes to the invention of slang.

"Overall, what slang in both medicine and psychiatry reflects is our own discomfort as providers with aspects of what we do," says Robert Klitzman. "Humour often covers awkwardness and discomfort."

He says the discomfort—which comes from uncertainty about the cause of psychiatric diseases, the effectiveness of treatments and the difficulty of studying the brain—gives rise to psychiatric slang.

Like the young intern Roy Basch in his novel *The House of God*, Dr. Stephen Bergman left an internship in internal medicine to become a psychiatrist. "What psychiatrists do does not have that basic foundation in reality," says Bergman. "In some few areas, like bipolar illness and in schizophrenia to some extent, you have some data on real interventions with drugs that work—very few, mind you. And very few when you take into account side effects, and even fewer when you find out that placebo works almost as well as every antidepressant in mild depression."

The result is that the whole profession, including the patients it tries to help, becomes stigmatized. You can see the stigma in the slang used by doctors to refer to their psychiatric colleagues.

As Peter Hukill and James Jackson catalogued in a 1961 article, it was common back then to refer to psychiatrists as head shrinkers, spooks and wig pickers. Such slang terms would almost never be used today because they would be regarded as overtly pejorative not just of psychiatrists but of their patients. However, a 2003 article in the journal *Ethics & Behavior* referred dryly to psychiatrists as members of the Freud Squad. I have certainly heard that one used recently.

The fuzzy science behind psychiatry creates diagnostic ambiguity that provides fertile ground for slang. In addition, the absence of solid scientific data means that the disorders listed in the *DSM* are constantly being revised and augmented. Between the first and second editions of the manual, the list of diagnoses increased from 106 to 182, while the third edition named 265. By the time *DSM-IV* was published in 1994, the volume had ballooned to include more than 300 disorders.

Many experts have criticized the growth of diagnoses listed in the *DSM*, often making the link between new illnesses and opportunities for pharmaceutical companies to make money. One such critic is Dr. Daniel Carlat, an American psychiatrist and author of *Unhinged: The Trouble with Psychiatry—A Doctor's Revelations about a Profession in Crisis*, published in 2010.

"The *DSM* and pharmaceutical companies have long been engaged in a symbiotic dance, with each partner supporting the other," Carlat wrote. "The proliferation of diagnostic labels has proved crucial for the growth of the pharmaceutical industry." Carlat says that while he believes in the value of certain drugs, when drug companies advertise a new cure for a condition, this benefits the APA because psychiatrists will buy the latest edition in order to objectify the treatment of their patients.

Bergman agrees. "In modern psychiatry, diagnosis is determined and written down in the *DSM* manuals," he says. "Who publishes the *DSM* manuals? The American Psychiatric Association. How much money do they make from that? Millions. Most of their money to support everything they do comes from the *DSM*. Everybody has to read it."

DSM-V—the latest edition—was released in May 2013. Its publication was mired in controversy, with extended debates about the inclusion and exclusion of certain illnesses. In fact, much of people's anger centred on the creation of categories many people wouldn't label as illnesses at all. In *DSM-IV*, bereavement excluded a diagnosis of major depression. But in *DSM-V*, the bereavement exclusion was lifted, enabling doctors to diagnose with depression patients grieving the loss of a loved one. In effect, grief and the depression that goes with it went from being just part of life to being a psychiatric disorder.

Resistance to the new order of things came from some unlikely sources. "Psychiatry is rapidly expanding and normal is shrinking," wrote Dr. Allen Frances, chair of the *DSM-IV* task force and a professor emeritus at Duke University in Durham, North Carolina, in an article in that appeared March 30, 2013, in the *Huffington Post*. "We need to rein in psychiatry and rein in the drug companies. We should get back to treating the really ill who need us badly and let people with everyday problems solve them with their own resources and resiliency—and not with a potentially harmful pill."

Klitzman doesn't think getting rid of the *DSM* is the answer.

"I guess it's tempting to see it as a necessary evil," he says. "However, I think the latest version could've been done better. I think they could've spent more time on making it better than they did, and field-testing it more."

///////

Given that the line between normal and psychiatrically ill patients is blurred, it's no surprise that psychiatric labels seem more like slang than words that define something important.

"It's difficult because another aspect of psychiatry is that it describes phenomena that one sees in people in everyday life," says Klitzman. "Take narcissism. People use the term *narcissism* [all the time]. It's part of common parlance. But in *DSM*, narcissistic personality disorder has clear criteria."

The psychiatric terms found in the *DSM* are supposed to be used to make a diagnosis. All too often, doctors—even psychiatrists—use such terms as *narcissist* not to diagnose but to label a patient. And when that happens, the diagnostic term becomes yet another piece of medical slang. I call that the weaponization of psychiatric labels.

Narcissism, called narcissistic personality disorder in the *DSM*, is a prime example. The word as it's commonly understood comes from a Greek myth about a boy named Narcissus who fell in love with his own reflection.

The *DSM*'s list of defining criteria for narcissistic personality disorder includes approval-seeking behaviour, a sense of entitlement and a predominant need for personal gain.

"*Narcissist* is a term that's thrown around a lot to devalue patients," Quinn says.

It turns out that the term can be used to devalue family members of patients as well. A resident says he remembers a male patient with an eating disorder who was having a lot of trouble accessing services. His medical condition made him ineligible for acceptance into a specialized treatment program. The young man attempted suicide, which led to him being admitted to hospital. The patient's boyfriend was a lawyer and, as his profession requires, he was wearing a suit when he came to the hospital to speak to the psychiatric staff about his significant other. "Oh, he looks pretty narcissistic," the resident remembers a member of the psychiatric team saying when he first saw the boyfriend.

The lawyer was advocating strongly on behalf of his partner, spouting suggestions and saying at one point that he was willing to call an influential business associate "Would it help if I spoke to him?" asked the boyfriend "Maybe he could get him into one of these programs. Maybe they could change the criteria."

When the team left the room, the accusations of narcissism returned, now with more intensity. "Wow, this guy's so narcissistic," one team member said. "I can't even handle this," said another. The resident was taken aback by his colleagues. "The reality is that this man's partner was in a lot of stress," he says. "Having an eating disorder is a high-mortality thing. It's not a joke. This patient was in a lot of trouble and the system was failing him. The lawyer was using every little thing he could find to try to help his partner, which I think anyone would ever want to do. But because he was advocating forcefully, they thought he had to be narcissistic."

I put the story to Dr. Robert Klitzman, the veteran psychiatrist. "I guess you can call that a kind of slang," Klitzman concedes.

The other diagnosis that often gets turned into a pejorative label is borderline personality disorder (BPD).

A senior medical student told me about a patient with advanced diabetes. The patient was in and out of hospital frequently. Her medications were being juggled in an attempt to improve her condition, but nothing was working. Her anxiety seemed to increase relative to her body's decline. She became very demanding.

One day, during rounds, a colleague of the med student presented the patient's history and current condition to the team. He had hardly finished his synopsis when the attending physician cut him off. "Oh," he said, "sounds like a borderline."

The student says there was no evidence that the patient had a personality disorder. "She was legitimately very stressed out about the impending end of her life," he says. The budding physician says the woman had gone through several doctors and many different treatments without feeling better, so she was appropriately distressed.

When the attending physician called the patient a "borderline," he didn't mean it as an additional diagnosis so much as a piece of slang to describe a patient who is frustrating her doctors.

Psychiatrists are generally more empathetic toward their patients than people like me are. But Quinn says even they will use the term *borderline* as a pejorative. Quinn was on his first rotation as a senior medical student when he heard a psychiatrist refer to a patient not by the formal term BPD but by borderline.

One doctor who isn't surprised that some psychiatrists use the term *borderline* as a piece of slang is Stephen Bergman.

"It's slang because the fact that such patients piss off even psychiatrists is the driving force to try and figure out how to deal with them," says Bergman. "It's pejorative because it's pejorative in psychiatry to a large extent, too. When I was starting out, nobody wanted to deal with borderlines. They were too hard."

Still, psychiatrists are relatively unlikely to use *borderline* as slang. Other mental health professionals aren't quite as reluctant. Sarah

Reynolds, the psychiatric emergency nurse, says she has referred to teenagers as "baby borderlines."

"You can't actually diagnose borderline until the person is 18 years of age," says Reynolds. "We'll say, 'This looks like a borderline.' It's like they're borderline-in-training. They're beginning their borderline career and they could either go one way or the other."

The fact that *baby borderline* exists at all is ample evidence of an adverse prognosis that justifies the term. And it's not the only term used to describe borderlines of a tender age.

"There's the teddy-bear sign," says Reynolds. "If someone comes in with a teddy bear, that's a borderline sign. And there's the suitcase sign. We always see that as a bad sign—someone who comes with the intent to stay for many weeks." Sometimes, the patient gets labelled with both slang terms. "People actually come in and sit the teddy bear down on top of the suitcase."

Some psychiatry residents at Dalhousie University in Halifax, Nova Scotia, told me they've heard *baby borderline* used there as well.

Terms like these are cruel and dismissive of teenagers exhibiting the early signs of BPD. Perhaps they indicate doctors' frustration and despair that a young patient is destined to be diagnosed eventually— and there's little or nothing even trained professionals can do to stop the course of their mental illness.

Still, Robert Klitzman believes there may be diagnostic value in using such slang: "Say an 18-year-old comes in clutching a teddy bear. There's something a little off about that. It's not specific diagnostically, but there may be symptoms and signs that have great sensitivity and specificity and others that are looser or suggestive or form a constellation."

Steven Bergman says the use of *borderline* as a label is due in part to the way BPD was formulated in the *DSM*. "The reason they're called borderlines is because it was a garbage category," Bergman explains. When he began his training in the 1970s, only two categories of psychiatric illness existed—psychosis (in Bergman's words, "really crazy people,") and neurosis ("people who were miserable but in touch with reality"). Everyone else was labelled borderline, because they bridged the border between the two.

Borderline personality disorder first appeared in *DSM-III*, published in 1987. "The fact that it is on the border of clearer definitional categories is a problem because it's being defined by what it's not rather than what it is," Klitzman says. "That's always going to be a problem because it suggests from the get-go that there's going be a lack of clarity about it."

Even a psychiatrist as seasoned as Klitzman says it's difficult to know when borderline is a diagnosis and when it's medical argot.

"It's not that precise," he says. "Given that some of the phenomena that led one to call someone a jerk or an asshole or a bitch are characteristics that one may also see in someone who [has] a borderline personality disorder, it's tempting to apply borderline personality more broadly. So, for instance, people are being described as being 'borderliney.' It's taking the verbal tools of psychiatry and using them to make sense of the behaviour, but also to put down people."

If a psychiatrist as esteemed as Klitzman sees the connection—not to mention the justification—for borderline as a slang term, there must be something to it.

⁄⁄⁄⁄⁄⁄⁄

During my interviews for the book, health professionals in just about every specialty named borderline patients as among the most annoying. They are also labelled by slang terms such as *splitter*, and are said to belong to cluster B or axis deuce (or axis two).

When a colleague tells me the patient I'm about to see is a borderline, what she's actually saying is, "Brace yourself. This patient is going to drive you up the wall."

Psychiatric nurse Sarah Reynolds says that "in the ER, people can get diagnosed as borderline after five seconds." Once, she overheard a doctor saying to his resident, "You can always tell when someone is borderline because they drive you crazy."

Emergency physicians routinely teach their residents that any time a patient provokes anger in the physician, the patient is probably a borderline. I've met colleagues who boast that they can diagnose a borderline on the spot. To me, that's dangerous to both the patient and the physician.

Las Vegas hospitalist Dr. Zubin Damania is one of the most caring physicians you will ever meet. Still, even he finds borderlines difficult to deal with. "These patients are some of the hardest to take care of," he says. "To half the staff they are super sweet and nice and pleasant, and to the other half they are absolutely nasty and vicious and evil, and often times those halves will switch within a day."

Damania says borderlines are nicknamed "splitters" because of their ability to split a medical team in two, pitting one side against the other. The categories cluster B and axis deuce reference the *DSM*'s organizational structure: using five axes or classes, the diagnostic manual attempts to group all of the various disorders and disabilities. Axis two encompasses personality disorders, including borderline personality disorder. "If someone has an axis two diagnosis, that usually means they have some kind of personality disorder that's going to overlay their care," Damania explains. "Borderline is a classic."

When Damania was an attending at Stanford Hospital in California, he cared for an axis deuce splitter. The patient was in her early fifties and suffered from severe high blood pressure and chronic pain. Her daughter had recently died of breast cancer, leaving the patient quite depressed. Believing her blood pressure to be danger-ously out of control, the patient's internist arranged for her to be admitted into Damania's care.

The patient decided Damania was a bad doctor. He says she made his life a living hell, but when her internist came to visit, she was sugary sweet. Much to Damania's disgust, the internist validated the patient's complaints about Damania.

Eventually, Damania had enough. "I understand you're not very fond of me," he said to the patient, "and that you're very fond of your internist." He felt compelled to offer to hand her primary care entirely over to the other doctor.

"Part of my ego structure in doing my job is that I tend to con-nect to patients very well," Damania says. "I have a pretty good bed-side manner. I can make people comfortable and feel at home and have a therapeutic presence that way." His inability to do this with the borderline patient frustrated him. When the borderline patient was nasty toward him, it was difficult for Damania not to be nasty in return. Psychiatrists call that counter-transference.

Damania's story reminds me of one of the things I appreciate most about being an ER physician. My involvement with patients is transitory. When I have a patient who is pushing my buttons, I almost always have an out: I can refer the patient to someone else. As a hos-pitalist, Zubin Damania doesn't always have that luxury.

////////

There is abundant evidence in medical journals that a psychiatric label isn't just pejorative: sometimes it can be fatal. Patients who present to a hospital with psychiatric complaints are less likely to be diagnosed, less likely to receive treatment and more likely to die much sooner than patients who do not have psychiatric conditions.

If anything, the gap in life expectancy between psychiatric and non-psychiatric patients is growing, according to a 2013 study published in the *British Medical Journal.* The study of more than 250,000 mental health patients in western Australia concluded rather shockingly that they lived an average of nearly sixteen years less than non-mental health patients suffering from the same medical conditions. Most of the deaths in the patients with mental health problems were due to undiagnosed and poorly treated cardiovascular conditions such as heart attack and stroke and cancer.

Another study published in *JAMA Psychiatry* in 2013 concluded that the death rate among psychiatric patients diagnosed with cancer is 30 percent higher than among non-psychiatric patients with the same types of cancer. The authors also found that psychiatric patients are less likely to receive specialized treatments for their cancer—such as surgery and chemotherapy—leaving tumours to metastasize.

I'm sorry to say that I have not only heard of this disparity in treatment, I have seen it with my own two eyes. During my training many years ago, when I was doing a rotation in internal medicine, my team was asked to see a patient complaining of severe pain on the right side of her mid back. The woman was about 70, and had been admitted to the psychiatric ward with a diagnosis of psychosis.

When we saw the woman, she was writhing with flank pain, a classic symptom of a kidney stone. The stone lodges in the ureter, a thin tube that carries urine from the kidney down into the bladder. The stone blocks the flow of urine, causing the kidney to become swollen with urine, which causes incredible pain. A sample of the patients' urine tested positive for blood, another telltale clue that the woman had a kidney stone that was scraping the inside of her urinary tract, causing microscopic blood to mix with her urine.

At the time, the standard way to diagnose a kidney stone blocking the ureter was to do an X-ray test called an intravenous pyelogram, or IVP. An X-ray technician injected some dye into the patient's blood vessel and then X-rayed her kidneys to see if the right kidney was swollen.

Both kidneys appeared normal, but the appearance of the right ureter suggested that the stone might have passed. The woman was still in pain, but instead of looking further, the team assumed that the woman was exaggerating her symptoms because she was depressed. We recommended that she take some painkillers. Mission accomplished, we crossed her off our list of patients to follow during their illness in hospital.

Three weeks later, an attending urologist (a surgeon who treats diseases of the kidneys, ureters and bladder) summoned us to the X-ray department to take a look at a second IVP that he had requested. During the ensuing three weeks, the woman had continued to suffer from flank pain, and the psychiatrist had asked the urologist for a second opinion.

When the urologist put the second X-ray up over a lighted view box, we looked at it in stunned, uncomprehending silence. The right kidney, which had appeared normal on the previous X-ray, was gone. It was gone, the urologist explained, because the woman did not have a kidney stone. She had a tear in the artery that nourished the right kidney. That had not only caused pain, it had blocked the flow of blood to the kidney, causing it to die. That's why the kidney was no longer visible on the X-ray.

The patient—whose rare condition might have been treatable when we first missed the diagnosis—died soon after.

Diagnosing problems like that is what people like me do for a living. The story of the woman and the lesson it taught me is something I try to keep in mind: even swallowers eventually get physically sick and die.

CHAPTER SEVEN

Caesarean Section Consent Form

The nursing station on the labour and delivery floor is throbbing with activity at 6 a.m. In the state-of-the-art birthing centre, banks of monitors—half of which have alarms going off—track fetal heart rates. The electronic bleeps are punctuated periodically by the sound of a woman in labour crying out.

Serena Fuzukawa, a second-year resident in obstetrics and gynecology (OBGYN), is handing over to fellow OBGYN resident Carl Young.

"You look like you've been to war!" says Young.

"G3P3 42-weeker three days postpartum with a PPH," says Fuzukawa. "She had a *very* successful home birth—until she started hemorrhaging, like three days ago. She arrived at 4 a.m. with a hemoglobin of 40 and a blood pressure of 60 over palp. I think we got all the RPOC out. She's getting blood and she's on IV antibiotics. Oh, and we saved her uterus."

"Sounds like a candidate for a Darwin Award," says Young.

"Nomination papers have been filed," says Fuzukawa. "Next, in birthing room 4, we have Rhonda Chan," 34-year-old 35-weeker, whiney primey, fourth visit. Not in active labour."

"Is she a diva?" Young asks.

"Just anxious," says Fuzukawa. "She's at two centimetres—exactly where she was the last three visits."

"Check her stress test and street her," says Young.

"Exactly," says Fuzukawa. "Amina Khan is just being brought in. She's G2P1, 36 weeks, BP 150 on 95."

"That was the puffy I saw on my way in!" says Young. "Am I sectioning her?"

"Nope," Fuzukawa replies. "She's NMD. Hutchison's on her way in to do it."

"Excuse me for having a Y chromosome," says Young resignedly.

"Don't mope," says his female counterpart reassuringly. "Tabitha Baker is G1P0 41-weeker with failure to progress. Let's see—presented with a carrot."

"Has she been pitted?" asks Young.

"Pitted, ARMed, frozen, which made her an ice cube. Now she's failure to progress."

"I assume I'm sectioning her," says Young.

"Talk to her doula first," says Fuzukawa. "They're still working on the lotus."

"I assume that's on the C-section consent form," says Young.

"Nothing like natural childbirth!" says Fuzukawa. She and Carl Young roll their eyes in unison.

/////////

The scene I just told you about is made up but the situations and the slang are not. Jargon and slang allowed Fuzukawa and Young to pile a lot of clinical information and some attitude into a short exchange. Let me unpack some of the highlights:

The first patient Fuzukawa talked about—the G3P3 42-weeker

three days postpartum is a woman who has been pregnant three times and has had three children, the most recent being born at 42 weeks' gestation (two weeks late) at home three days earlier. A PPH stands for a postpartum hemorrhage. A hemoglobin of 40 translates into 40 grams per litre, roughly one-third of a normal blood level. A blood pressure of 60 over palp is slang for 60 systolic, well below a normal blood pressure of 120 over 80—indicating severe shock.

As Fuzukawa explained, the woman arrived in shock. Thanks to the doctors' quick action removing the RPOC (retained products of conception—bits of placenta still inside the womb), plus blood transfusions and intravenous antibiotics, they were able not only to save the woman's life but her uterus so that she'd be able to have more children.

Darwin Award is obstetrical slang for a woman who chooses to have a high-risk birth at home—far away from a hospital with its life- and womb-saving doctors and equipment. It's a reference to the annual Darwin Awards given to individuals who carry out colossally stupid or foolish acts that usually end in death.

Fuzukawa referred to Rhonda Chan as a whiney primey—slang for a woman who keeps coming to the Labour and Delivery ward because she thinks she's in labour when she isn't. *Whiney* is slang for anxious, while *primey* refers to the fact that the woman is a primp, or primipara (first pregnancy). The cervix dilates during labour to make way for the baby. At ten centimetres, it is fully dilated; at two centimetres, the cervix is nowhere near ready.

Young asked if Fuzukawa is a diva. That's OBGYN slang for a woman who keeps complaining about being in labour in the hopes that her doctor will perform a Caesarean section and get the whole thing over with.

Next up was Amina Khan. With a blood pressure of 150 over 95, Khan has pregnancy-induced hypertension. The normal blood pressure during pregnancy ranges from 110/70 to 120/80. *Puffy* is a slang term used by OBGYNs to say the woman's face is swollen and her complexion is grey—both subtle indications that she has pre-eclampsia, a condition during pregnancy associated with high blood pressure. Left untreated, it can cause seizures and threaten the lives of mother and child.

One of the main treatments of pre-eclampsia is an urgent Caesarean section; that's why Young asked if he would be sectioning Ms. Khan. Fuzukawa's reply that the patient was NMD was a deal-breaker for Young: it stands for "no male doctor," an increasingly common request.

Tabitha Baker's story is filled with jargon and slang. *Carrot* is slang for the fact that the configuration of Baker's cervix meant that a vaginal delivery was unlikely. *Pitted, ARMed* and *frozen* meant that Baker had been given the IV drug Pitocin to make her womb contract forcefully, her membranes had been ruptured (ARM stands for "artificial rupture of the membranes") to induce labour, and she had been given an epidural (frozen) to reduce her pain. Unfortunately, the epidural had frozen Baker so well she stopped being in active labour—hence the reference to ice cube.

Baker has a doula, a non-medical person who provides support to the mother before, during and following delivery. The reference to lotus is not slang per se. A lotus birth is the practice of leaving the umbilical cord uncut after birth so that the baby is left attached to the placenta until the cord separates naturally after a few days. Lotus birth—once rare in Western culture—has become increasingly popular among proponents of natural childbirth. In this case, *working on the lotus* was code for saying that Baker—supported by her doula—was reluctant to agree to a Caesarean section.

The reference to Caesarean section consent form was pure slang. It's a subtle dig at birth plans, which are favoured by proponents of natural childbirth as well as by mothers who want to control almost every aspect of the birth. It was coined by OBGYNs on the assumption that of all the procedures that can take place during a birth, a Caesarean section is just about the last one a mother-to-be with a birth plan would ever consent to.

The slang enabled Fuzukawa and Young to share a great deal of information with lightning efficiency. Moreover, it reflected the ever-present tension found on the labour and delivery ward. I'm not an OBGYN, but what struck me was just how much latent and manifest tension was packed into such a spare conversation: tension between mother and OBGYN; tension between OBGYNs and midwives and doulas; tension between male OBGYNs and female patients; tension between family doctors and OBGYNs; tension between different worldviews of pregnancy and birth; tension between the close proximity of happy endings and unspeakable disasters.

Looked at in that way, OBGYN slang is a critical safety valve that defuses the tension and permits people under conditions of extreme stress, fatigue and sleep deprivation to work and function together.

Still, the tension is always there. It's been that way for a long time.

///////

Today, the Tabitha Bakers and Amina Khans of the world come to hospital to have their babies. A hundred years ago, they would have had their babies at home. Whether they and their babies would have survived back then is a pertinent question. Changes in where and how babies are born have led to changes in language. Understanding the tension produced by those changes is key to understanding OBGYN slang.

The transfer of childbirth from homes to hospitals gave rise to many medical procedures that have since been judged unnecessary.

A family physician who has practised low-risk obstetrics for twenty years and who is deputy chief of family medicine at a hospital in Toronto says that in the 1950s, for instance, "every woman, that's *all* women, needed an episiotomy to create extra room whether they needed extra room or not. And forceps on the baby's head to protect the fetal head."

An episiotomy is a surgical cut in the perineum, the skin and underlying tissue roughly between the vagina and the anus. Today episiotomies are known to heal poorly and to cause loss of bowel movement and bladder control and are used only if the baby is in distress or the woman is at risk of tearing. Forceps were used in conjunction with episiotomy to pull the baby by the head from the woman's body.

All this snipping and pulling came from a popular notion that babies could be harmed as they travelled through the birth canal. Today we know better. "There's no part of the female pelvis—vagina side wall, even ischial tuberosities (the bones along the birth canal)—that harm that baby's head," says the family doctor.

Rosanne Gephart, a certified nurse-midwife in Santa Rosa, California, believes the motive for some of the extra work involved in birth is financial. "A lot of money is made off the complications of birth," Gephart says. "The physicians and the anesthesiologists—everybody—make more money when things are complicated."

In 2010, 98.5 percent of births in Canada took place in a hospital, according to Statistics Canada. During the same year in the United States, the number of hospital births was slightly higher, at 98.8 percent.

The shift from home to hospital also means a shift in who is attending the birth. Formerly the domain of midwives and family doctors, births are increasingly being attended by OBGYNs.

In 1986, 43 percent of American family physicians performed

deliveries, compared with 28 percent in 2006, according to the American Academy of Family Physicians.

One of the reasons family physicians have moved out of obstetrics "could be the obstetricians' faults," says Dr. Shiraz Moola, an OBGYN in Nelson, British Columbia. "If we assume that we're the best at doing this, that nobody else can do as good a job, then we may push family physicians out. And I don't think that's ideal."

Moola believes "a family physician is an optimal specialist to provide good care. You know they're looking after you through your pregnancy. They very well may have looked after you through your infancy and your childhood. They may look after you as you get older in life."

A few family doctors still do deliveries, and they love their work. "I'm what's called a birth junkie," says one family physician. "It never goes away, the high that you get from having that baby."

Dr. Gerry Prince, director of the Family Medicine Maternity Clinic in Medicine Hat, Alberta, offers a couple of different explanations for the exodus of family doctors from maternity care. "One is the time commitment. The inconvenience of the on-call requirement," he says. "The other would be training and competence and confidence. Today's residents aren't permitted to be on call as often as we used to be. Which means they can't get as much experience doing obstetrics. Obstetrics and other procedural things are mostly experience based: you have to do enough to feel good."

When Prince was doing his family-practice residency, he did 100 deliveries on his own. Now, he says, residents are lucky to do as many as twenty.

While family doctors may continue to be absent from maternity wards, there's evidence to suggest that midwives are on the rise. In the United States, the number of births attended by certified nurse-midwives more than doubled from 1989 to 2002, rising to 7.7 percent from 3.3 percent of all births, according to a study published in the *Journal of Midwifery and Women's Health*. Since then, the numbers have held relatively steady and are expected to increase.

Who does what during a delivery has a profound effect on how it's done and what language is used to describe the process. "There's a fundamental philosophical difference in approach to obstetrics between obstetricians and family docs [and other] low-risk obstetrics people, whether that's midwives or whoever," Prince says.

And there are political differences.

A family doctor who does low-risk obstetrics at an urban hospital learned all about such differences a few years ago. At the hospital where the family doctor works, one of his patients—a healthy woman with no medical complications—was booked for a C-section. During morning rounds, the family doctor leaned over to the OBGYN scheduled to do the operation and said, "My patient is the 10 o'clock Caesarean. I just want you to know that she's normal and healthy."

The OBGYN became visibly upset for several reasons. Having been trained to expect complications, he wasn't about to buy the family doctor's assertion that all was well with the mother-to-be and the baby. More important, by informing him at the last possible moment, the family doctor was telegraphing to the OBGYN that he didn't need his opinion as to the situation. In effect, the family doctor was calling upon the OBGYN to just do the C-section, turning the OBGYN into what's known in the business as a C-section technician. And that really makes OBGYNs bristle.

"Why am I hearing about this now? Why didn't I get a referral a week ago?" The OBGYN screamed at the family doctor.

The family doctor was taken aback. "This is very routine surgery," he thought to himself. "You could do it in five minutes if you had to."

The OBGYN's chief, the family doctor's chief and the two physicians had to sit down to sort out the incident. They patched things up, but not before the family doc learned an important lesson about how OBGYNs feel about the work they do.

"Surgeons do not want to be seen as Caesarean section technicians. They do not want to be seen as residents in house for the family doctors in the office," the family doctor says, "and managing that relationship is a serious challenge."

In telling me this story, the doctor revealed an important bit of slang for OBGYNs: *C-section technicians*. They're also called baby catchers. These terms are hated by OBGYNs because they diminish the scope of what they are capable of and provide insight into why relationships between those who provide maternity care are at times strained. Family doctors tend to be less interventionist than OBGYNs. More than that, both are fighting to hold territory in the labour and delivery ward.

Part of this battle for territory includes "privileging," a formal process in both Canada and the U.S. through which family doctors apply to hospitals to be allowed to do uncomplicated obstetrics. These seemingly polite requests for permission are often laced with the underpinnings of a high-stakes political turf war: the more procedures doctors can do, the more money they make.

Another primary-care doctor who does low-risk obstetrics has also had his share of turf battles. Previously, he had been used to a routine of family doctors granting privileges to their peers. But the region where he worked was amalgamated with another and the new region did it differently. There, the department of obstetrics decided who got to do what, and its selection process proved more contentious. The GP remembers asking the chief of the obstetrical department if family doctors could have the right to manually remove placentas—a life-saving procedure in certain instances. In a perfect world, after the mother gives birth to the baby, she pushes out the placenta and the uterus contracts to close off all the blood vessels inside. If, however, the placenta stays put, the vessels will continue to bleed and the woman is at risk of a postpartum hemorrhage. Manually removing a stubborn placenta—called a retained placenta—is one way of avoiding such a scenario.

"No, I don't think family docs should be able to do that," the chief said. "I don't think they do it safely."

"I have people who have been [removing placentas] for twenty years and you're telling me that you wouldn't privilege them?" the family doctor asked.

"I just don't think they should," was the reply.

"So if I've got a woman who's delivered and is bleeding and needs a manual removal, and I can perform that service, I should let her bleed and call the obstetrician and wait for them to come in the middle of the night?"

"Yes," the chief said, "you should wait. If the patient bleeds to death, it's not your fault. You didn't have privileges."

I find that shocking: Putting patients at risk because you're unwilling to share responsibilities with a colleague is unconscionable.

Family doctors aren't the only ones likely to call obstetricians butchers or C-section technicians; midwives also wage war with OBGYNs.

"I remember it was often like having to get over the perceived hostility that the OBGYN is being called in, and that leads to a C-section," says a GP who completed a four-year residency in obstetrics and gynecology before switching to family medicine. "There was a kind of a sense [coming from midwives and their patients] that all the OBGYNs want to do is cut, that we didn't really care about patients. We didn't really care about the moms or the babies, and that we didn't get that birth is a natural process. The message we got from them is that the midwife really cared and really wanted the mom to have a natural delivery and that the OBGYNs were kind of the enemy to that."

The former OBGYN resident remembers one instance in which the patient (of a midwife) was in early labour that was not progressing well. The woman's contractions began to peter out. The baby's fetal heart rate showed a pattern known as late decelerations—which means the heart rate went down late during a contraction and stayed down after the contraction ended—a sign that the baby was in distress and at risk of asphyxia.

"I'm consulted to come and talk about starting oxytocin to increase the contractions of the woman's uterus and to speed up the labour," the former OBGYN recalls. "The woman is very hostile to that idea because she wants to have a natural delivery and not a C-section."

The former resident says she'd often feel the tension as soon as she walked into a patient's room.

"There's a body language of a barrier—like a defence—starting," she recalls. "I would see the frown. I'd see them almost squaring for battle like they're thinking they have to protect their baby and protect their vaginal delivery—like I was this person who was going to try and take it away from them—and turn it into a C-section."

Nancy Hewer, a perinatal nurse in British Columbia, explains why the relationship between an OBGYN and a midwife might be adversarial: "You see very different styles of practice between an obstetrician and a midwife. A midwife is more . . . encouraging of the woman. [She allows] the woman lots of time to get through the process, whereas obstetricians—lots of nurses, as well—just sort of say, 'Well, we've got to make this much progress in this amount of time.' I think there are system pressures in terms of budget-centred care instead of patient-centred care." In budget-centred care, Hewer explains, the focus is on moving the new mother out of the hospital as fast as possible so that someone else can take her spot.

Sometimes, the lines between these models of maternal care aren't so clear-cut. "In reality, you can find family-practice physicians, especially, who really want to practise like a midwife," says Rosanne Gephart, the certified nurse-midwife. "And you can find midwives who practise like physicians."

Gephart's comment reminds me of another slang term: *medwife*, or a midwife whose practice aligns more with the medical model than it does with that of her midwife colleagues. Among midwives, it's used pejoratively as a way of saying the midwife has abandoned her roots for the medical model. When OBGYNs use it, however, they're implying the midwife is infringing on their territory.

OBGYN Shiraz Moola says, "These are midwives who think they know better than the OBGYN about when to deliver or how to deliver a patient." He says that midwives are sometimes referred to as frustrated obstetricians.

Gephart says that, for some midwives, practising within the medical model is more a matter of necessity than it is choice: "If you've got six patients in labour, and your job is to prove to the obstetrician who's on call that each one of these people is making progress and going to have their baby and not need surgery, then you manage them in a very medical fashion," she says. "You're still a midwife, but you are performing obstetrics. When you're putting on internal monitors, when 90 percent [of your patients] have epidurals, can you really still call yourself a midwife? You can. You're just a different kind of midwife."

Midwives working within a hospital and abiding by hospital rules might threaten OBGYNs if they feel their role is being usurped and their skill set relegated to the confines of the operating room. Midwives who avoid hospitals altogether, however, can pose a different kind of frustration.

"I probably bear them less goodwill," Moola says. "We've sort of made attempts to bring them in from the cold and try and engage these individuals. I've seen moms come in here with their placenta hanging out between their legs, and oftentimes they've been abandoned by those same individuals who were helping guide them through their pregnancy. Part of it is because [the midwives] recognize if they walked into the hospital they may be facing sanction or legal summons."

///////

The history of birth gives rise to obstetrical slang as well as to the medical jargon heard every day in delivery rooms—much of which irks health-care providers, especially midwives. I'm talking about words and phrases that at first glance might seem benign—to doctors. *Delivery, incompetent cervix* and *unproven pelvis* are a few examples.

When birth moved from the home to the hospital, having a baby became more about the doctors overseeing the process than about the labouring mother. Rather than the mother *giving birth*, the obstetrician was *delivering her baby*. The two phrases describe two profoundly different experiences.

The family doctor I spoke to who is currently the deputy head of family medicine at a major urban hospital in Toronto says he remembers the first time he witnessed a child being born. "I donned a 'space suit,' or full surgical greens, including mask and cap," he recalls. Like her doctors, the soon-to-be mother was also covered up. She was fully draped with a surgical cloth. "All you saw was surgical drape [with a] little hole in the middle," he recalls.

Wide-eyed, he watched as a tiny head emerged from the "little hole in the middle" of the draped cloth. "There's no woman. There's no patient. There's no father. [And there's] probably epidural anesthesia, so no sound," he says, thinking back. You can see how in this scenario, *delivery* is the only word that makes sense.

As more and more births took place in hospitals, the birth-is-risky-business attitude took hold. With it came language. *Unproven pelvis* is an example of a phrase that was probably not thrown around much in farmhouse bedrooms, but nowadays is frequently heard in hospital hallways.

"[It's] coming from that risk perspective," says perinatal nurse Nancy Hewer. "'We just don't know if this baby's going to fit through that pelvis. We just don't know until we give it a try,'" she says, mocking those who use the term.

Incompetent cervix is another term often attributed to the rise in hospital births. When a woman's cervix starts dilating prematurely and she's unable to carry the pregnancy to term, she's said to have an incompetent cervix, a phrase that makes many in maternity care recoil. "I think it's a loaded [phrase] just in terms of the woman," says Hewer. "She hears, 'Okay, so you've lost your baby. You have an incompetent cervix.' The issue around the language for me is: Just how is it taken in by the woman? And how is she then perceived? And how does she perceive her body?"

Dr. Marjorie Greenfield is a veteran obstetrician-gynecologist with more than twenty years of experience. She's a professor at Case Western Reserve University School of Medicine and at MacDonald Women's Hospital of University Hospitals Case Medical Center in Cleveland, Ohio. "The term 'incompetent cervix' always was to me the worst," she says. "I think the new term is 'cervical insufficiency.' Whether that's much better, I don't know."

Not everyone thinks this area of obstetrical jargon is worth dwelling on. "Call a rose whatever you want to call it, just stick to whatever it is," Gerry Prince says. "If we would spend more time on being able to roll with things and not be offended by every little nuance of whatever language we're using, then all of us would be a lot better off."

For Greenfield, it's the attitude behind the language that needs addressing. "Fixing the language without talking about the attitude isn't going to do anything. Then you're just changing the language in order to be politically correct," she says.

Not that the language is changing all the quickly or all that much. If you want proof, look no further than the birth announcement of His Royal Highness Prince George of Cambridge, first-born son of Prince William and Catherine, Duchess of Cambridge, on June 22, 2013: "Her Royal Highness The Duchess of Cambridge was safely delivered of a son at 4:24 p.m."

When it comes to the British monarchy, it's hard to argue with tradition, no matter how outdated the language seems to be.

///////

Midwives and doctors alike will tell you that the great tension between them is largely about how they view birth itself. Midwives say it's a normal process; doctors say it's risky business.

"Up until the moment the baby is out, you never really know if things are going to go sideways," Shiraz Moola says.

During moments like these, slang is invented on the spot. Moola was once called to a delivery room where a mother was giving birth to a breech baby, an infant who is entering the world bum first as opposed to head first. Optimally, the head—which is the widest part of the baby's body—comes out first to widen the birth canal. Having the head come out last increases the risk it will become trapped, and the baby will asphyxiate. Fortunately, breech babies occur in only 3 or 4 percent of all deliveries. While most breech babies are delivered through Caesarean section, in the right hands a vaginal birth can be just as safe.

Normally, during a breech delivery the baby's buttocks will

appear first, with the baby's back lined up against the mother's pubic bone. In the case Moola was dealing with, the breech was turned sideways.

It was not a position Moola had encountered before, but it was too late for a Caesarean section. Moola delivered the baby's feet and moved the baby so that its spine was in the proper position. Then came the next challenge: one of the baby's arms was stuck. Normally, the arms fall down; in this case, he had to rotate the baby 180 degrees to allow for both arms to come out.

"But then I couldn't get the head out," Moola says. "And that oftentimes is the one moment that scares the pants off OBGYNs. Because literally you have minutes in which to deliver the child or it will suffer a lack of oxygen to the brain. So I lengthened the [umbilical] cord a little bit and I could feel that the pulse was fairly weak, but again what happened is the baby's head turned sideways. And I didn't know any manoeuvre for that."

At this point the mother was screaming so loudly the anesthesiologist could barely hear Moola when he asked him to give the patient nitrogylcerin, a medication used to relax the uterus.

"No doubt my heart was going at 180 beats a minute," Moola says. The drug worked and the OBGYN was able to turn the baby's head so that it lined up with the rest of the body. The baby was born alive and without having suffered any damage. Moola now calls that one last turn of the baby's head a Hail Mary manoeuvre.

It's moments like these that make many believe that birth is dangerous. You never know what could happen and you best be prepared. "That's the very reason a lot of physicians won't go into obstetrics," Prince says.

Moola has another nickname for situations where a Hail Mary manoeuvre might be necessary: he calls them Matrix moments. "Time and space slows down and there's this intensity of focus where you're completely oblivious to everything else," he says. Usually, these moments last a matter of minutes, but they feel hours long. If there's a lot of blood, Matrix moments are sometimes called bloodbaths or change-of-underwear moments. The last one comes from situations so messy the blood has soaked through the OB's surgical greens.

Moola remembers walking in on a colleague's particularly bloody Matrix moment.

Moola arrived at a hospital to begin his shift. The maternity ward is normally a zoo, with nurses and doctors bustling from one room to the next. But that night, it was completely deserted. Standing at the main desk, Moola spied a trail of blood starting at the doorway of a patient's room and leading all the way to the OR. "It looked like someone had taken a body and dragged [it] down the hallway," he says.

Moola followed the trail to the operating room, where he opened the door and looked inside. What he saw looked like "some kind of tableau that you might see in a Renaissance painting of something out of Dante's *Inferno*," he says.

"There was essentially the entire staff—a whole bunch of nurses, a whole bunch of obstetricians and doctors—surrounding this mom, and it looked like a bomb had exploded in the room." The mother was suffering a prolapsed uterus, meaning her womb had fallen from its normal position into her vaginal area. It "can be a catastrophic complication," explains Moola. "The mom suddenly goes into shock and then begins to bleed like stink."

The obstetrician had his hand up to his forearm inside the woman's body in an effort to help massage her uterus back to its proper size and muscle tone. The staff stood frozen around him, waiting to see if his efforts would work. They did, and the woman was saved from bleeding to death.

"That to me would be a very vivid memory of the amazing things that can happen in terms of the risks of childbirth," Moola says.

A family doctor who does low-risk obstetrics agrees. "Birth is normal, natural and healthy, and it's all just beautiful in a dark room with all of us humming 'Kumbaya'—until something goes terribly wrong," he says.

At the same time, Moola recognizes that problems like a breech baby or a prolapsed uterus are the exception rather than the norm. "I think it's rare that things go from normal to absolute chaos," he says.

It's the medical model's attachment to rare complications that makes some OBGYNs uncomfortable. "We're looking for problems," Marjorie Greenfield says. "There's almost this internal logic that leads you down a road where you do a lot of interventions that lead to a lot more interventions that lead to a lot more interventions that lead to a C-section and then everybody thinks, 'Oh, well, you know, boy, good thing she didn't deliver at home because she needed a Caesarean.'"

The derivation of the term *Caesarean section* itself is fascinating. According to *Cesarean Section—A Brief History* (published by the U.S. National Library of Medicine), the term derives from Roman law under Caesar, which decreed that all women who died during childbirth were to be cut open in an attempt to save the child "for a state wishing to increase its population." The notion that the term is derived from the surgical birth of Julius Caesar has been dismissed, because Caesar's mother Aurelia is believed to have lived long enough "to hear of her son's invasion of Britain."

Ironically, Greenfield says, the slang *C-section technician*—the term that that made the OBGYN yell at the family doctor—may be deserved. "I think what we do is, often—we manage the labour in such a way that we paint ourselves into a corner and then we have to cut ourselves out of it."

In addition to slang, adages are being coined to describe the phenomenon of too much intervention. "They say that the most dangerous place for a woman in early labour is Labour and Delivery," an OBGYN resident says.

The belief that interventions are necessary promotes a culture of fear, another aspect of modern maternal care that has many up in arms. "I think we terrify our mothers from the first prenatal visit," says a family doctor. "And we keep them scared until it's all over and [then we say], 'Oh, you've got a beautiful, healthy baby. Aren't you the happiest lady in the world?'"

Perinatal nurse Nancy Hewer says malpractice lawsuits contribute to this culture of fear. The threat "would obviously influence anybody's practice," she says.

A doctor who practises in the U.S. was faced with exactly the kind of situation Hewer is talking about. It began with a prolonged labour, or a patient's "failure to progress."

In these scenarios it's become common practice to induce labour after twenty-four hours of waiting. One reason for doing so is to avoid an infection called chorioamnionitis, which occurs when bacteria from the vagina enter the womb. It can lead to serious complications for both mother and child, including the death of the baby.

The doctor chose to wait for labour to come naturally. The mother showed no signs of infection and when eventually they decided to induce her labour, all seemed to still be going according to plan. It wasn't until an hour before her delivery that the signs of infection showed up. The doctor delivered a baby who was acutely infected, severely ill and eventually brain damaged.

Situations like these are a doctor's worst nightmare. Not only do doctors grieve the loss of the patient, but they can be tied up in litigation for years. OBGYNs have learned that it's better to deliver a healthy baby by whatever means available than to open the door to disaster.

There's tension between health professionals and the views of birth they hold to be true. Then again, there's tension between doctors and moms to be—which is revealed by some telling slang.

Not infrequently, Dr. Moola says he is summoned to repair an unassisted home delivery gone wrong. He told me about a woman who had fired her midwives because they weren't passionate about her birth plan—which was to deliver at home in a location that didn't have road access.

The birth didn't go as planned. When the mother called the hospital for help, Moola persuaded her to come to the hospital and she ended up having a vaginal delivery, but her waters had been ruptured for a few days and she ended up with an infected uterus and a postpartum hemorrhage. "I put my hand inside to remove her placenta and by this point she'd already lost a litre of blood," says Moola. "And as I removed her placenta—one keeps their hand on the uterus to get it to contract—I just feel the uterus essentially just give up."

Moola says they rushed the woman to the OR, where they worked furiously to try to stop the bleeding. In the end, they had to remove her uterus in order to save her life.

As heartbreaking as situations like these are, the frustration of doctors at having to manage catastrophes that could have been avoided leads to slang. Scenarios like these sometimes get labelled as natural selection at work, free-to-die births or bleed-to-death births.

"The decision to have an unassisted home delivery is akin to landing an airplane by reading about it. You know you'll get on the ground, but you'll probably end up in pieces," Moola says. He notes that one of the greatest factors contributing to maternal mortality around the world is the lack of a skilled birth attendant.

On the other side of the spectrum are whiney primeys or divas. A whiney primey is a woman in her first pregnancy and in an early phase of labour who comes to the hospital day after day, believing she's ready to have her baby when she isn't. The former resident in OBGYN said she saw patients like that all the time. She says she felt sorry for them. "In my head I'd be thinking 'You think this hurts? Just you wait until labour happens.'"

Dr. Gerry Prince invented his own slang to describe whiney primeys. He calls them "perineophobes," derived in part from perineum, the part of the body between the pubic bone in front and the tailbone in the back, where a vaginal delivery takes place. The *neo* part of *perineophobe* means it's the woman's first time in labour, while the suffix *–phobe* refers to a phobia or persistent fear of an object or situation.

"I use this to refer to women who are so sensitive to any touch or pressure in the vaginal area that it can actually prevent or delay a vaginal delivery," says Prince. "The first clue in the delivery room is that when you do the first examination on a woman who thinks she's in labour, you can barely complete a vaginal examination without her crawling off the bed!"

Prince says that for most women the urge to push during the second stage of labour is enough for them to overcome whatever discomfort or apprehension about discomfort they possess. Perineophobes are different. "They just can't do it," says Prince. "They will make all sorts of noise, turn all shades of red and purple, tense all sorts of other muscles to satisfy nurses, doctors and family members that they are trying. But every time the baby's head descends a little, they back off. It is worse, of course, without an epidural. Most women you can coach through it, but sometimes you just can't! Sometimes, they pretend to push until they are exhausted and end up a going for a C-section."

That's assuming they reach the second stage of labour still determined to have a vaginal delivery. After three or four visits to hospital, many such women want the pregnancy over and done with.

"They say, 'This is too much. I just want to have a section,'" says the former obstetrics resident. "It can be a long, drawn-out process, especially for the poor women who have that niggling really early labour for days, which can exhaust anyone. I had a lot of empathy for those women," she adds.

To section or not to section is a major source of tension in labour and delivery wards these days. In 2010, the Caesarean delivery rate in the U.S. was 32.8 percent of all births, according to the National Center for Health Statistics. While this percentage is high, it actually represents the first decline since 1996. From 1996 to 2009, the C-section rate rose nearly 60 percent.

No OBGYN I spoke to says he or she does C-sections on demand. Most see the high rate as the natural extension of the argument in favour of managing risk. But not everyone agrees.

"Maternal mortality in the United States is going up. And I think there are two explanations for it," says Marjorie Greenfield. "I don't think that our care has changed tremendously. I think the explanations are that obesity increases your chance of maternal mortality, and having had a previous Caesarean increases your chance of mortality."

There's wanting a C-section and there's dictating the terms under which the operation—and all the other procedures that often go with it—take place. Not surprisingly, there's a slang term for that.

"A princess is a woman who wants her epidural the minute she enters the hospital," says the former resident in obstetrics. "A princess phones ahead and says 'I'm coming. Have the anesthetist on standby for my epidural.' There's no question that they love their baby, but on top of their brain is the cosmetics of the situation. When they have a C-section, they dictate how many centimetres they want the incision to be."

The upside of a smaller incision is a smaller surgical scar.

Unfortunately, the downside of a smaller incision is that there's less room to get the baby out. Sometimes, the incision is so small that the baby's head can get stuck, a condition known as skin dystocia.

"Several times [during residency], I saw that there wasn't room to bring the baby's head up through the incision," say the former OBGYN resident. "Mid C-section, we'd have to negotiate with the woman to extend the incision."

Closely related to a princess is a diva. "My favourite was one of my patients who literally almost had her baby in the parking lot because she had to get her makeup on," Gephart says.

////////

Medical birth professionals of all stripes agree on one thing: their mutual disdain for birth plans. A birth plan is a document written by a woman to describe how she would like her labour to go. Some of them run several pages long.

Moola and colleagues call a multi-page birth plan by the slang term *Caesarean section consent form.* Recognize the sarcasm here: For whatever reason, be it scientific or chance, women who show up with birth plans tend to have labours that go anything *but* according to plan. If it says "no C-section," they'll probably end up needing one. If it says "I don't want an epidural," they'll probably end up begging for one in a moment of intense pain. If it says "I want my husband to cut the umbilical cord," he'll probably end up stuck in traffic when the moment comes—or passed out on the floor of the birthing suite.

Almost everyone I interviewed for this chapter confirmed the irony. "I usually tell them, don't bring a birth plan because it's like the kiss of death," Prince says. "Anything you put on there that you don't want to happen is going to happen, so just don't make a birth plan."

More than that, Moola says, women who come in with detailed

plans often end up getting what he calls the "full-meal deal," or the whole obstetrics package—epidurals for long periods of time, induced labour and forceps included. Oh, and they get the worst complications.

Greenfield thinks there may be a scientific explanation for the positive correlation between birth plans and complications. "I think there's a kernel of truth in that the more anxious someone is, the more they try to control their experience in the hospital by making a birth plan as if it were a contract. And the more anxious you are, the less well labour goes," she says.

Birth plans can contain items that some would think of as eso- teric—for instance, to have a favourite song played over and over again during labour.

"I can think of one woman wanting to labour while on her hands and knees with chanting music in the background," the former obstet- rics resident recalls. "The only pain control was to be deep [Lamaze] breathing, with absolutely everybody in the room taking part in the breathing: the nurse, the midwife, the doula and the resident."

Some birth plans require that health-care professionals obtain the approval of the patient's clergy before intervening. In some cases, it's not a spiritual leader but a doula who the woman in labour grants the right of refusal.

A doula is a non-medical person trained to assist and support a woman, her partner and her family during pregnancy and childbirth. Although there are many training programs for doulas, they tend to be as brief as one or two weekends. There may be little if any profes- sional oversight of the work they do.

The former resident says that on several occasions, the birth plan stipulated that the woman's doula was to be consulted before any obstetrical intervention. One time stands out in her mind. The woman was in the late stages of labour when the baby's heart rate showed signs of fetal distress. As a consequence, the woman's midwife called in the obstetrical team to assess the situation.

"There were problems with the fetal heart rate," the former OBGYN resident recalls. "There's a predictable pattern of fetal distress and a predictable course that if you let that go long on enough, the baby's most likely going to die."

Both the attending and resident in obstetrics concluded that an emergency C-section was needed to get the baby out before oxygen deprivation led to irreversible brain damage. They explained things to the mother-to-be, but she said to clear it with the doula.

"Mom was saying, 'Oh, I don't know,' and the doula said, 'No, the baby's fine. Keep with on with the labour,'" the former resident recalls.

As time went on, the fetal heart rate kept dropping—an ominous sign. The former resident says she and her attending kept suggesting a C-section with ever-increasing urgency. "The mom kept turning to the doula and saying, 'What should I do?' And the doula's saying, 'No. You can still hear the heartbeat,'" the former resident recalls. "Then it was 100 and then it was 80, then 60. I still get tingles thinking of this. We're just standing in front of the mom saying, 'We are losing this baby and we have to go.' Then, the heart rate was 40, and then 20. Finally, the doula just kind of nods. We race down the hall and do the C-section to get the baby out.

"I always wonder how that baby did in the end" she says. "I can't help but think that there's brain damage of some sort because of waiting all that time."

The former resident is almost shaking as she tells the story. "I'm angry for the mom, for the baby and angry for the system," she says. "I don't know what led to that mom to not trust the medical advice and [instead] trust this person who had a weekend training course about supporting moms."

Some women put a lotus birth on the birth plan. A lotus birth is a practice in which the umbilical cord is left uncut following the birth—leaving the baby attached to the placenta until the cord separates at the baby's umbilicus several days later. The practice is common in some parts of the world. Until fairly recently, it was all but unheard of in North America—but has become quite trendy of late. The placenta may be placed in a bag with pine cones and herbs and spices—and even diamonds—to reduce the smell as the placenta tissue decays.

"The placenta is to be kept, and there's a spiritual ceremony said over the placenta," says the resident. "And then they take the placenta home and plant it under a tree."

There are no obvious health benefits to leaving the newborn attached to the placenta for the up to ten days needed for the umbilical cord to detach. In 2008, the Royal College of Obstetricians and Gynecologists (RCOG) noted that if left for a period of time after the birth, "there is a risk of infection in the placenta which can consequently spread to the baby. The placenta is particularly prone to infection, as it contains blood. Within a short time after birth, once the umbilical cord has stopped pulsating, the placenta has no circulation and is essentially dead tissue." The RCOG strongly recommended that babies whose mothers opt for a lotus birth be monitored carefully for any signs of infection.

Gephart says she's had women come in with birth plans drafted by their attorneys. Others have theirs laminated. Gephart calls these red flags. "Red flag means this is somebody you're not going to stick your neck out for," Gephart says, "because they've already shown themselves to be either unreliable or unappreciative."

Gephart isn't alone in thinking women with birth plans are unappreciative. "Part of being an obstetrician is the belief that you know what's best for this person in this particular moment," Moola says. "And that's sometimes hard to juxtapose with a mom who may honestly feel that there's something else that needs to happen."

Oftentimes, a birth plan is unnecessary because it forbids procedures such as enemas and shaving of the pubic hair—things that fell out of favour years ago and are no longer done.

Some doctors and midwives are fighting back. Greenfield told me about one obstetrics department in Cleveland that doesn't allow birth plans. They tell potential patients, "You have to trust us. If you don't, go find another doctor."

OBs think of birth as a medical procedure—something proposed and formulated only by doctors and other health professionals. It's unheard of, for example, to come into the hospital with a plan for how you'd like your appendectomy to go. In an OB's mind, the same goes for birth.

Greenfield says a birth plan is a list of preferences, not a contract: "You can't really have a birth plan because you don't know what's going to happen."

One family doctor says he tells expectant women that "no part of this is plannable or knowable. You have wishes that I could try to respect. We'll call those birth wishes. I dissuade my patients from being invested in [birth wishes], because I'm not loving the disappointment after."

Sometimes, birth plans evoke even stronger reactions among health professionals.

"I've seen a nurse rip one up," perinatal nurse Nancy Hewer says, adding that she thought the nurse was being disrespectful. She tries to reframe the discussion. "To me it says, 'Okay, this is somebody that I really need to spend some time with to establish trust and really let her know that I'm listening to her.'"

///////

Arguably, one of the biggest changes in maternal care inside the hospital has been a near total gender swap.

I can remember when it was almost impossible to find a female OBGYN. Today, not only do women outnumber men in OBGYN residency programs, it seems strange to see a male physician in the role.

"Sometimes people have come in and left the hospital when it's only males on call," says a male OBGYN resident who is training in the U.S. "They'll go to another hospital, shopping for a female obstetrician. Or they'll ask to be transferred out as high risk by ambulance, because there's only male obstetricians on. Not only do people not want obstetricians anymore, they definitely don't want male obstetricians. It's a bit disconcerting, as young residents that are wanting to have a long career, to be rejected like that so flatly."

The change has led some to question the role of male physicians in the field altogether.

"Sometimes people look at them a little funny, like they're somehow a bit perverted and that they went into the field so that they could look at female vaginas all the time," says a former female resident in OBGYN. "When I've talked to my previous male colleagues, I think that was really hard on them. It reflects a misunderstanding about the field."

The female resident thinks there's a lot less overt sexism in medicine. But she says she's encountered a more subtle kind of sexism directed by female attending OBGYNs against female residents.

"I think the OBGYN residency is one of the hardest on the residents, and the least forgiving on pregnant residents," she says. "I remember one woman went into early labour during a shift when she was a junior resident. She's thirty-two weeks pregnant and starts to have contractions. She's afraid to ask to stop working because you just don't do that. Finally, she's kind of crippled by these contractions. Some of the other residents who are working with her go to the attending on that night and say that she's got to go home because she's in labour.

"And the attending says she can't go home because she's on call. And if she goes home, she's going to have to make up the shift! We'd never treat a patient that way."

The trend towards mostly female OBGYNs appears irreversible. According to a 2008 report by the Society of Obstetricians and Gynaecologists of Canada, 84 percent of OBGYN residents are female, 16 percent male.

If and when the last man is driven from obstetrics, I seriously doubt that will end the tension between doctor and patient.

CHAPTER EIGHT

Incarceritis

A 28-year-old man I'll call Roger is brought to the ER by the police. Roger had been charged with possession of cocaine for the purposes of trafficking. As the charges were being laid, Roger had started complaining of chest pain, which prompted the trip to the ER. Two female police offers brought him to the ER; both were smirking at me as I introduced myself to the patient.

"What seems to be the trouble today?" I asked Roger.

"I've got pains in my chest. They're going down my left arm. I think I'm having a heart attack."

Roger then proceeded to answer yes to every textbook question related to heart disease: yes to having shortness of breath, yes to having high blood pressure, yes to having a family history of heart disease, and so on. Around the fifth or sixth yes, it dawned on me that Roger had boned up on the symptoms of a heart attack. I decided to ask him one I was sure he hadn't read about.

"Do your ears ring when you pass water?" I asked Roger. He looked puzzled and unsure of how to answer. After about twenty seconds, inspiration came to him.

"Doc, now that you mention it, that's exactly what's been happening," he replied.

Now it was my turn to smile. Roger had answered yes to something called the positive functional inquiry test, a bit of medical slang an attending physician taught me when I was a student. A functional inquiry—also known as a review of systems—is a series of questions designed to get further details about the presenting symptom and a fuller picture of the patient's overall health. A functional inquiry is exhaustive, yet useful only when it yields information that is both pertinent and true.

As my teacher explained, some patients get confused by these questions and answer yes to each one because that's what they think the doctor wants to hear. The devious ones—patients like Roger—answer yes each time because they think that's the ticket to receiving a diagnosis. Whenever he became suspicious, my teacher said, he would ask patients if their ears ring when they pass water because this bogus symptom has no basis whatsoever in medical fact.

"I'm not worried that you're having a heart attack," I reassured Roger. "Just to be on the safe side, let's do an electrocardiogram and get some blood tests."

Later, when I finished my night shift and was handing over the ER to a colleague working the day shift, I told him about Roger.

"I love patients with incarceritis," he said. "Move 'em in and move 'em out."

///////

Roger's story is inspired by hundreds of encounters with patients in police custody. *Incarceritis* is the medical argot my colleague learned as a resident to describe the conditions of people in jails, prisons or any other kind of police custody who fake symptoms to earn a trip to the hospital. The creator of incarceritis took the verb *incarcerate*, added the suffix *–itis*—Latin for inflammation—and created a delightful yet totally fictitious noun. As a piece of slang, it's witty enough to get high marks from *The House of God* author Dr. Stephen Bergman.

"Ah, yes, I've heard that one," says Dr. Jeff Keller, a former ER physician who now is the medical director at not one but several jails as well as juvenile facilities in Idaho. "When they're arrested, before they come to jail, they get it in their heads that if they can be sick enough, we'll have to release them. They'll seize upon anything in their pointy little heads that makes them sick enough to get out of jail.

"Diabetics, especially type 1 diabetics, can manipulate their blood sugars and there's very little that you can do to stop them if they really want to have their blood sugar go high or low. For example, in the jail we will draw up their insulin and hand it to them to inject. They'll turn slightly away from us and inject the insulin underneath their clothes or onto the floor, so their blood sugar goes sky high and then we have to take them to the ER. Conversely, they'll take their shot of insulin and then refuse to eat, causing their blood sugar to crash, which again means a trip to the ER."

Keller's experiences both as a jail doctor and an ER physician have given him a unique understanding of medicine inside and outside of the correctional system. "There are a lot of differences between correctional medicine and regular medicine," says Keller, who writes the blog *Jail Medicine*. "In a family practice, and a little less so in the ER, basically you believe everything the patient tells you. But in corrections, we always have to view all of those health claims kind of skeptically. They may be truthful but what they say may also be a means to an end."

And that is the essential difference between Keller's outlook on patients and mine. I assume patients are telling the truth; hard-fought experience has shown Keller and those of his ilk otherwise. In Keller's world, when it comes to patients who are convicted criminals, truth telling is at best a fifty-fifty proposition. In general, inmates who work a con on the doctors and nurses who work at correctional facilities are looking for one of or a combination of drugs, sex, power and influence.

Often, though, they're just looking to make life behind bars a bit more pleasant—like getting out of work detail. ER doctors and nurses may call it incarceritis; the health professionals who work inside those sliding prison doors call it the *whine line*. That bit of slang, which is listed No. 13 on scrubsmag.com's "Top 47 Slang Terms Nurses Use," refers to "inmates who suddenly need to see medical because it's raining and they don't want to go to work. In the hospital they are the uninsured that show up in the ER with sniffles, etc."

Prison inmates work as part of a rehabilitative labour program. The Thirteenth Amendment to the U.S. Constitution permits penal labour as a punishment for a convicted criminal. Detainees who have not been convicted cannot be forced to participate in such programs.

In the ER where I work, I may get one or two requests a shift for a medical note excusing a patient from work or school. A whine line is that multiplied by twenty or thirty—in a prison no less! You don't have to remind Dr. Mike Puerini of that particular challenge. Puerini is a physician at the Oregon State Correctional Institute, a medium-security prison in Salem that houses 800 inmates serving sentences of one to fifty years.

It's hardly surprising that some prison inmates use illness or disability to get out of work duties. Puerini says the biggest complaint he has with the whine line is not with inmates; it's with correctional officers who ask doctors to validate claims by inmates for everything from time off work to providing a wheelchair.

"The officers say they've got these fifty guys who don't want to work today," says Puerini. "They bring each one up to the doctor, and the doctor has to decide who has to work and who doesn't have to work. In my opinion, that's an officer not doing his or her job. Somebody's got to say no.

One of the reasons Puerini doesn't want to validate the health claims of inmates any more than he has to is just how easy it is to get fooled by a good story. If you believe every word prisoners say, you won't last as a corrections physician.

"We had this doctor," Puerini recalls. "I love this guy. He's one of my favourite people, but he drove me crazy while he was working in the building. He saw working in this prison as an extension of his Christian gospel way of life and I'm the last person to fault that. But he was happy to give away the farm because he saw it like his mission work and other charitable work."

/////////

There's a strong connection between the prison MD who fears giving in to inmates on the whine line and the ER doc who fears giving in to patients who are pretending to be ill to score a prescription for narcotics. But there's one big difference. Prison docs know what ER staff can only suspect: that their patients are criminals with hidden agendas.

The polite term we use for this heterogeneous group of patients is *drug seekers*. But that's an awfully wide net. They range from people who are addicted to the drugs they covet to criminals in the business of acquiring prescription drugs to sell or barter. Some are bona fide patients who got turned onto narcotics by GPs or specialists with little time to take a proper history and not much else to offer in their therapeutic toolkit.

The thing is, it doesn't seem to matter to us what kind of drug seeker a patient happens to be. We treat them all with a dollop of contempt that, to an outside observer, is shocking. The mere act of importuning, wheedling and sometimes pleading for drugs just seems to bring out the worst in us.

"We use varying degrees of profanity for them," says the ER nurse at a community hospital in Kansas who blogs under the name Not Nurse Ratched. "We'll say, 'Douche bag over here is demanding Percocet again.' Or 'We've got a bunch of barefoot hillbillies in there that want their hillbilly heroin.'"

Hood Nurse, the ER nurse who blogs about her experiences at *Adventures of Hood Nurse: Hood Hospital*, says she and her colleagues call drug seekers trolls.

"One in particular had a major medical problem at one point but has been out of the woods since," says Hood Nurse. "She'll come in for various complaints and want to get [the narcotic pain reliever] Dilaudid for whatever complaint it is, regardless of how ridiculous it is. She'll say she's allergic to everything but Dilaudid."

Hood Nurse and her colleagues have another slang term for narcotic seekers. They say the patient has ADD—not attention deficit disorder (a legitimate medical condition) but something more on point. "It stands for Acute Dilaudid Deficiency," says Hood Nurse. "Somebody comes in for various complaints and they keep adding more on top of the pile. And they've had a thousand other visits this month for other vague complaints."

Dilaudid is one of the most powerful prescription narcotics in the painkilling arsenal. It can be given in pill form. In the ER, I give Dilaudid in its intravenous form to patients with severe pain caused by broken bones, kidney stones, acute abdominal problems and a host of other painful conditions. Dilaudid has long been known among drug seekers as "drugstore heroin" because, when shot intravenously, it produces a heroin-like high.

"You'll ask your colleagues what's wrong with them and it's like 'Oh, you know, they've got ADD,'" Hood Nurse says, her voice dripping with sarcasm. "They're coming in just because their 'serum Dilaudid levels' are low."

That slang is a pun on a bona fide kind of medical treatment. We measure chemicals such as sodium and potassium because your body needs them to run properly. We don't measure serum Dilaudid levels. If a patient is in severe pain, we just give the patient a shot. The slang term *serum Dilaudid level* suggests the patient thinks she needs Dilaudid more than we think they do.

Troll, douche bag, ADD. Not Nurse Ratched says her ER colleagues sometimes say the drug seeker is suffering from *percoceto-penia*—a made-up bit of slang that means the patient is suffering from a lack of Percocet, a narcotic tablet of which addicts and recreational users have long been fond.

Nurses aren't the only ones who have it in for drug seekers. Just ask Dr. Donovan Gray, an ER physician and the author of *Dude, Where's My Stethoscope?* The book, a collection of stories about Gray's experiences as a doctor, devotes not one but two chapters to his experiences with drug seekers. "Anyone who's worked in an ER knows about drug seekers," writes Gray. "They're those incredibly annoying chuckle-heads who are forever trying to con us into giving them prescriptions for certain drugs. OxyContin is their Holy Grail, but Percocet, Dilaudid, fentanyl patches, or just about any narcotic will do."

A colleague who works in another part of Canada recalls a young woman who used to visit an ER complaining of migraine headaches. The thing about migraine is that you can't see it on a CT scan of the head. Either you believe the patient or you don't. The woman had visited the ER five times in seven days and each time had received a shot of Demerol—another powerful narcotic. After the fifth time, as she walked out the sliding doors, a nurse shot at her: "Why don't you come back when you have a *real* cause for your pain?"

The woman—who also had a psychiatric history—took the

nurse's suggestion to heart. She left the ER, walked to a nearby second-floor bar with a balcony and jumped, cracking both of her heel bones and two vertebrae in her back. As paramedics wheeled her back into the ER, the woman again demanded Demerol, which she got immediately; unlike a migraine headache, her broken bones gave her an obvious and legitimate source of pain.

What strikes me about the episode was not just the disdain shown for the patient but the brazen way the doctors and nurses involved in her care laughed as they told the story. They were even chuckling as paramedics wheeled her in—as if delighted not just at having a good story to tell but that the drug seeker took their advice and became a *real* patient—one with three broken bones, all self-inflicted.

There are many reasons drug seekers elicit a disdain bordering on hatred. For one thing, they're seen as freeloaders. "That's a blanket term that people in my hospital use not just for the drug seeker but the social services seeker or 'whatever-else' seeker—the people that come in and immediately make a thousand demands," says Hood Nurse. "They want a cab voucher. They want footsies [soft foot covers that doctors and nurses wear over their street shoes when they go to the OR]. They want a sandwich. Healthy ambulatory people who are there for a minor complaint can easily provide these things for themselves. But freeloaders know these things are available and they demand them—usually in an obnoxious fashion."

ER nurses are often quicker than doctors to label freeloaders and for a very good reason. I might see the patient only once, so I don't see the pattern nurses catch because they work more hours than we do. Of course, it helps that, unlike physicians, my nursing colleagues don't have to make the call and decide whether a patient is legitimate.

The second reason for all that contempt has to do with the fact that some drug seekers—though not all—have PhDs in lying. The doctor-patient relationship is based on trust. You trust that I have the knowledge and the skill necessary to take care of you. I trust that you're telling the truth. There's no scanner that reveals whether you're really in pain. The fact is, you could be lying about it and I probably wouldn't know the difference. I have to trust you.

Like most medical or nursing grads, I entered practice believing every patient tells the truth. When I was just starting out and I saw an ER patient writhing on a stretcher with what she said was terrible pain in her back, I believed her. I ordered a shot of a narcotic to relieve the pain. When she felt better, I sent her home with a prescription for thirty tablets of Dilaudid. As she left, she thanked me for being a kind and caring physician. I felt good about myself. A few weeks later, a police officer paid me a visit. He showed me a list of fifty or so doctors who had given the same woman scripts for narcotics within days of each other. All of us had been duped by a bogus patient—a con artist.

When that happens, some doctors worry that authorities will take their medical licence away. That seldom happens, unless you're a total rube who falls for every drug-related scam under the sun. Still, some physicians feel like they've been burned. I suspect the thing that gets most of us is the role reversal from the usual doctor-patient relationship. We're used to having an overwhelming edge on our patients in terms of knowledge and experience. CT or MRI? Chemo or radiation? How the heck is a patient supposed to match wits with us?

In the world of drug seeking, the roles are reversed. The drug seeker—a con artist with a nose for a doctor's psychological weak points—is the suave professional. And the doctor, more often than not, is the vastly outmatched dupe. The dilemma for doctors on the front lines is that the patient whose story sounds legitimate might be a well-rehearsed, lying con artist. Or he might look like a criminal but be telling the truth. Or maybe he's a little of both.

I know a lot about drug seekers because more than twenty years ago, I was one of the first ER physicians to become fascinated by "drug diversion"—the movement of legal narcotics and other controlled substances (the ones controlled by government legislation) from regulated professionals such as physicians and pharmacists to the street. I've written articles and book chapters and have given hundreds of lectures and workshops on how to recognize drug seekers. Long before actor Hugh Lawrie said it on the TV show *House*, I was teaching colleagues how to be lie detectors.

To me, there was always something deliciously refreshing about the idea that book-wise yet emotionally dumb MDs could be out-foxed. In some ways, I've always enjoyed pulling people's legs by telling a good fib myself. Besides, there was a gap in our education. I could not find a single textbook that paid any attention to drug seeking. That lack attracted me.

In the politically correct world of hospital medicine, you're not allowed to be pointedly contemptuous with even the most difficult of patients—unless they're drug seekers. I suspect it's appealing for many of us to be able to disrespect patients we don't understand and certainly don't like.

"Most seasoned ER docs come to automatically suspect malingering whenever unknown patients present with symptoms of this ilk," writes ER colleague Dr. Donovan Gray in *Dude, Where's My Stethoscope?* "This attitude is unfortunate, because it undoubtedly causes us to treat some bona fide sufferers with less compassion than they deserve."

To Dr. Stephen Bergman, a psychiatrist by training with a long career treating patients with addiction, the attitude seems all too familiar. Back when he was inventing medical slang in the 1970s, one dreadful acronym was already in use by health professionals: SHPOS, for sub-human piece of shit. "It seemed even too cruel for us, but it was New York, you know," Bergman recalls. "That was cringeworthy."

Berman says SHPOS was used to refer to the criminals, drug addicts and gang members who frequented Bellevue Hospital Center, a well-known and well-respected psychiatric facility in New York City. "When an alcoholic or a drug addict comes into the ER and is going to die but you know how to save him, you know it's going to take a lot of work," says Bergman. "But you also know that you'll see him back next week. It makes you so angry at these people. You've spent your whole life getting trained to save people, and these people seemingly don't want to save themselves."

///////

Like the ER physician or the GP who gives drug seekers whatever they want, it's easy for a doctor to get a reputation in prison as an easy mark.

"If you're an easy mark on the inside, word travels fast in our small town of 900 convicted felons," says Puerini. "To work in a prison, you have to be smart."

One woman who long ago figured that out is Nicole Donaldson. For eight years, she worked as a nurse at the Vancouver Island Regional Correctional Centre in Victoria, British Columbia. The facility was called the Saanich Prison Farm when it opened back in 1913—so-named because it's located in the District of Saanich, which is named after the Saanich First Nation. Although renovated in the 1980s and '90s, the correctional facility retains its Edwardian-era brick façade and courtyard. Donaldson says the whine line is alive and well at Canadian correctional facilities.

"We had that a fair bit," Donaldson recalls. She says inmates complained of back aches or pain from injuries sustained in motor vehicle accidents, to get prescriptions for narcotics. Some said they had anxiety to get Lorazepam, a sedative. Try as they might, the inmates she saw never got a thing from her. "They usually went to the softies," Donaldson says in reference to her more empathetic colleagues. She says many convicts also complained of toothaches. She acknowledges that a lot of them probably had tooth pain—much of it due to illicit drug use. For instance, methadone is known to cause dental decay.

"I wasn't very sympathetic because the pain was self-inflicted," she says. "It wasn't like we held them down and made them do that. I never ever caved on anything. *Never.*"

Occasionally, a clever inmate would set up a more elaborate scam to get drugs. Donaldson says some inmates injured themselves deliberately to earn a trip to the local ER. "They'll break their own finger so that they can go to the hospital because their girlfriend's going to leave them some coke or something in the toilet paper roll on the second floor in the bathroom by the ER," says Donaldson. "If they put that energy to work [on the outside], they'd be millionaires."

Donaldson says she was rarely fooled because she learned a valuable lesson from a nurse I'll call Brad. She says Brad told her that "if I learn nothing else from him, to please learn that if their lips are moving, they're lying."

Donaldson says she didn't follow Brad's advice blindly. "I would go and research those requests for pain meds," she says. "Almost 99 percent of the time it was all lies. So you kind of get tainted."

///////

A 2006 study by the U.S. Bureau of Justice Statistics found that nine out of ten inmates with mental illness abuse alcohol or drugs. So it's hardly surprising that much of the lying that Brad taught Nicole Donaldson about involves the acquisition of drugs or alcohol.

Jailhouse booze is known as squawky or pruno; whatever you call it, it's a mash made from water, bread (for its yeast content) and fruit.

"It smells horrible," says Jeff Keller. "So most of it is caught because the deputies or correctional officers smell it and track it down."

When it comes to drugs, sooner or later, many of the drug seekers who plague ERs get caught forging scripts, robbing pharmacies or committing other crimes to pay for their drug habit and end up in jail or in prison. Many are addicted to narcotics such as OxyContin; correctional physicians put these inmates through a detoxification program to get them off narcotics. Occasionally, inmates continue to receive regular doses of a narcotic for chronic pain or they receive methadone (a synthetic narcotic that's given to ward off withdrawal symptoms) as part of a drug-maintenance program.

Those exceptions aside, narcotics simply aren't given out very often. Inmates will look for any medication with mood-altering or sedating properties that can be used as a substitute for their drug of choice. Jeff Keller says antidepressants including doxepin, amitriptyline and trazodone are favourites. So is the over-the-counter antihistamine Benadryl. Inmates can use these drugs. If they're really clever, they can sell them to fellow inmates.

At the Wilkinson Road Jail in B.C., Nicole Donaldson says, inmates traded drugs such as methadone and Seroquel, also known as Quetiapine, which is prescribed for psychotic symptoms. It is also prescribed as a nighttime sedative for elderly patients with dementia who have a tendency to get agitated. "They'll trade any kind of medication," Donaldson says.

Also in demand are Ventolin puffers—also know as inhalers—which contain Ventolin and Salbutamol and are prescribed to patients with asthma. Inmates believe that, when snorted, Salbutamol produces a speed-like effect. "We have to be very strict on puffers because those little monkeys will spray medication onto a counter, scrape it off and then snort it," says Donaldson. "They will snort anything that can be crushed."

Trading drugs in prison takes some planning. Instead of prescriptions, inmates receive their doses one pill at a time and are watched as they swallow. Some use quite ingenious methods to hold the drug in their mouth while pretending to swallow it. Inmates and the doctors who look after them call that "cheeking."

"You can hide it in your cheek, but there's a lot of ingenious ways of doing it," says Keller. "There's sleight-of-hand, like a magician; you palm it so it never gets into your mouth. One inmate used the space where he was missing a tooth to hide pills. Inmates also use denture adhesives like Fixodent placed high up on the roof of the mouth to hide pills. If we really wanted an inmate to take his pills, we would crush it and watch him take the crushed medication. But Keller knows one inmate who would stick a crushed pill on his tongue, pretend to swallow it, then scrape the pill fragments and saliva onto a piece of paper and mould that into a ball, let it dry and then sell it.

"Inmates are really good at cheeking their pills," says Keller. "I suspect we only catch about one in ten. A lot of the time, we only learn about it because an inmate has some sort of adverse drug reaction tied to a particular pill. But they aren't supposed to be taking that pill, which means they got it from another inmate. So we see who else in their dormitory takes that particular pill. Sure enough, once you confront them with the evidence, they confess."

Nicole Donaldson says that when she worked with inmates, the nurses would crush tablets into a paste, add it to food and watch the inmate eat it. It was foolproof—or so the nurses thought.

"I had a fella come up to me at the jail and ask if I could get him on some Seroquel 25 milligrams," she recalls. "He said it really works. I asked him how he knows it works. He said he'd been taking it for two months."

When Donaldson checked the inmate's file, she discovered he hadn't been prescribed Seroquel, which is used to treat the symptoms of schizophrenia and other psychotic disorders. She tracked the inmate down in the prison yard and confronted him about where he got the drug. Turns out the seller was a fellow inmate who swallowed the paste, vomited it up onto a piece of paper, let the vomit dry, then sold the dried effluent. Donaldson asked the man how he could stand swallowing the fellow inmate's barf. "I'm selective about who I buy it from," she says he told her.

Donaldson recalls that another inmate who was prescribed methadone while incarcerated managed to throw up the drug into a condom and sell that.

///////

Some inmates are motivated to get drugs; some want light duties or time off work. Others still want to charm corrections employees. Inmates call that "downing the duck." It's a slow, painstaking process by which prisoners recruit and seduce correctional staff to do their bidding.

Not surprisingly, prison nurses and doctors are frequent duck-hunting targets.

"Inmates talk about the word *grooming*," says prison doctor Mike Puerini. "They groom one of the people who work for the prison to get what they want from them. They learn a secret about one of the people who work in the prison. Then they hold it over that person's head and extort them for pills or sexual favours. They get [prison staff] to share personal information like how their kids are doing. They engage them in conversation about their personal life. Once you start, some of these guys are pretty bright about human nature. They can see when you're having a bad day."

Nicole Donaldson says she, too, has seen inmates manipulate health professionals. "There was an RN that was railroaded out because she was too kind and too touchy with them," she says. "She was an okay nurse but she was a bleeding heart. When the boys would give her a story, she would buy it. So then it caused the rest of us grief, because she would do these nice things and the rest of us wouldn't."

Donaldson says that, in rare cases, it was corrections officers and other support personnel who cultivated relationships with the inmates. "We had a female officer that would come on nights and she would do aerobics in a mental health ward." Until staff realized she was exercising within sight of the inmates, "we couldn't figure out why the boys all got excited and caused her grief all night."

Prison employees who get involved with inmates aren't committing minor indiscretions, says Mike Puerini. "We've had situations in Oregon in which health-care workers have gone to prison because they've had physical relationships [with prisoners]. It's especially difficult for health professionals, because a lot of them are women working with men prisoners."

And it's not just about getting drugs or sexual favours. In some cases, corrections officers have helped prisoners escape. But those are extreme examples. In health care, we teach students about maintaining tight boundaries with patients. Outside prison, it's all about professionalism; inside, it's often about keeping health-care workers safe.

Puerini says he once was getting ready to leave on holiday when, "about a week before I left, I saw an inmate who wished me a nice vacation in Hawaii. I was pissed off because somebody let this guy know that I was going to Hawaii. Well, guess what? I don't want this guy to know I have a family, much less that I'm going to Hawaii. Now he can call his buddy on the street and tell him that Puerini's going on vacation and see if you can find his address.

"You always have to have it in your brain," says Puerini. "If you don't, you're going to let down your guard and when you do, you're going to put people in danger."

It's drummed into every medical student and resident that relationships with patients are strictly forbidden. It's ridiculous to have to say that goes double when the patient is a convicted criminal. That it ever happens is evidence that some health professionals have psyches that are quite wounded.

//////

The prodigious capacity to tell whoppers is but one thing that separates patients behind bars from the ones I see in the ER. Another is the way jail-bound patients use their anatomical attributes for nonmedical purposes that can be quite profitable.

Jail doctor Jeff Keller set me straight on those who use various orifices to smuggle contraband into correctional facilities. People not familiar with the correctional system use *jail* and *prison* interchangeably. But there are some important differences between the two. In the U.S., jails are most often run by sheriffs or a local governing authority and hold people awaiting trial or serving short sentences. Prisons, which are operated by a state government or by the Federal Bureau of Prisons, are for convicted criminals who typically serve longer sentences. In Canada, jails are run by the provinces and their inmates are serving sentences no longer than two years less a day. Canadian prisons, known as penitentiaries, are run by the federal government.

As far as smuggling is concerned, in the United States, the Supreme Court has ruled that it is illegal for officers to do a body-cavity search on people admitted to jail unless there is probable cause; in prison, such searches are permitted. As a result, people going to jail frequently use body cavities to smuggle everything from drugs to personal items to weapons. Not surprisingly, the medical slang used to describe such activities is rather crude.

"Inmates refer to that as keestering if it's in the rectum and cootching if it's in the vagina," says Keller. "I've also heard it referred to as the prison locker. We doctors call it the pink purse and the brown purse. You can put anything you want in the pink purse and the brown purse and the Supreme Court says that we can't look for it.

"Inmates can secrete an amazing variety of things. One woman was caught with a compact case of makeup, a methamphetamine kit that included a syringe and a little vial of meth, a cellphone and a hard pack of cigarettes [in her vagina all at one time]. That was pretty impressive.

"There was another inmate who wasn't caught until he stabbed another inmate with a steel rod that was eighteen inches long and sharpened to a razor point that he had smuggled in the brown purse."

Not surprisingly, a lot of the pink- and brown-purse stories involve the smuggling of drugs and related paraphernalia.

"We had a guy come in with cocaine up his backside," Nicole Donaldson recalls with unconcealed delight. "The man was processed and then transferred immediately into the segregation part of the jail. There, he was placed in a dry cell; the water in the toilet system had been turned off to prevent drugs—and everything else—from being flushed away. Every single time he has a bowel movement, they go through the stool. And then they shine a flashlight up his backside to see if there's more coming. They took eight balls of cocaine out of his backside. And a crack pipe."

Few stories can top that of Christie Dawn Harris, a 28-year old dealer in crystal methamphetamine from Oklahoma who reportedly hid a .22-calibre handgun loaded with three live bullets and one spent shell in the case—all inside her vagina. A story in the *New York Daily News* in March 2013 said that Oklahoma police found the gun after arresting Harris during a drug raid. The story goes on to say that officers found bags of meth shoved up her anus. After pleading no contest to possession of methamphetamine with intent to distribute, gun possession and bringing contraband into jail, Harris was sentenced to twenty-five years in prison for her crimes.

Recently, a case made the news that tested not only the constitutional powers of the police but the role of doctors in police work. According to a news report by the *Knoxville News Sentinel*, in February 2010, Felix Booker and his brother were stopped by police as they made their way through Oak Ridge, Tennessee. Catching the aroma of marijuana, the police booked the suspects for felony possession. At the police station, investigators did a strip search. Suspecting that Booker had secreted cocaine in his rectum, police asked him to consent to an invasive search. Booker agreed; however, Dr. Michael LaPaglia, the doctor who carried out the search, found that Booker clenched his buttocks during the search. The doctor then injected Booker with a drug that paralyzed him and then intubated the suspect to protect his airway. Dr. LaPaglia repeated the invasive search and found 10.2 grams of crack cocaine in Booker's rectum.

Booker was convicted of possession of crack cocaine with intent to distribute and was sentenced to five years in prison. However, in August 2013, the Sixth Circuit U.S. Court of Appeals overturned his conviction because the paralysis, intubation and anal search violated Booker's Fourth Amendment rights. The court said the police "effectively used LaPaglia as a tool to perform a search on Booker's person."

///////

With health professionals like Nicole Donaldson and Jeff Keller, you get the sense that, in a perverse way, they admire the ability of inmates to secrete contraband in a rectum or vagina. But as keen observers on the front lines of prison or jail culture, they know quite well that this sort of behaviour has a very serious side.

A 2010 study by the National Center on Institutions and Alternatives (NCIA) found the suicide rate in county jails to be three times that of the general population. Despite a decrease in the overall rate, suicide continues to be a leading cause of death among people in custody.

And it's not just inmates with suicidal thoughts who are at risk of premature death; incarcerated individuals in general are five times more likely to have mental health problems. Donaldson says she looked after inmates at Wilkinson Road Jail with mental health problems, including bipolar affective disorder, as well as issues related to drug addiction. One of Donaldson's duties was to give prisoners their regular doses of antipsychotic medications.

Part of Donaldson's hardened view comes from the fact that on more than one occasion she's had to stare down an inmate who was threatening her.

"One time, I walked into segregation where inmates are housed in little matchboxes the size of your bathroom," Donaldson recalls. "That's where they are locked up when their behaviours are inappropriate." A prisoner yelled obscenities at her. "They were absolutely the most vulgar words I've ever heard in my life and I said to the officer, 'I want him charged.' That sent a wave through the jail that you don't mess with this nurse."

That's when Donaldson discovered something else about prisoners. She's good with them because she can get inside their heads.

"I have a son with ADHD [attention deficit hyperactivity disorder] and I've been surrounded by people who have acting-out behaviours," says Donaldson. "I didn't realize how much I loved behaviours until I was at the jail for a little while."

By behaviours, Donaldson means assaulting fellow inmates

with makeshift weapons, screaming, even rioting. One day she was on duty in segregation when a riot broke out in a large common area the size of a hotel lobby. "You could feel the energy in that room. I swear that the room was breathing," she says. "The boys were chanting and banging on the doors. All of a sudden it's lockdown. I'm standing there and about eleven officers in black riot gear come busting through the door. I'm thinking to myself, 'This isn't a movie. Back up!'"

After the riot was put down by armed police, Donaldson stood calmly as the inmates were escorted out the door of the room, popping antipsychotic pills into the mouths of most of them as they walked by.

Many of today's inmates are quite used to popping psychiatric meds. Nearly 15 percent of male offenders and an astonishing 30.1 percent of female offenders have been admitted previously to a psychiatric facility. The widespread use of antipsychotic medications has helped to fuel the deinstitutionalization of psychiatric patients—which in turn resulted in the closing of many psychiatric facilities. In the absence of community supports, these psychiatric patients inevitably act out; in the absence of a psychiatric bed, they tend to be prosecuted through the criminal justice system.

Some say cutbacks to welfare entitlements are also a factor in the incarceration of people with mental health issues. A former social services worker says she saw first-hand the devastating effects that cuts and being thrown out of the system to fend for themselves had on patients: "I had the experience of being cornered a few times in the office by raging and ranting clients with mental health issues, one of whom actually was wearing a tin foil hat to ward off the voices. It was so sad and such a shame that so many end up in the prison system because of their displacement and having nowhere else to go."

Since 2002, the United States has had the highest rate of incarceration in the world. According to the Bureau of Justice Statistics, in 2011 the number of prisoners in state and federal correctional institutions was just under 1.6 million. Many have substance abuse issues and have never taken good care of their health.

"I think we're up to about 40 percent of my patients have some chronic health problem," says prison doctor Mike Puerini. "They've got high blood pressure, diabetes, cholesterol and hepatitis C. I had a guy who had a heart attack last year."

And the prison population is getting a lot older. According to the Oregon Department of Corrections, in 2012 the state had 674 prisoners older than 60, up from 258 a decade earlier. A budget report by the state's Legislative Fiscal Office blamed the increase on mandatory minimum sentences and other changes in sentencing policy.

"Young healthy guys make a mistake," says Puerini. "Except that now, my average population is in the forties and fifties. I've got people in their sixties. I've taken care of people in their eighties."

Puerini even had one patient live long enough under his care to develop dementia. "In Oregon, because they get a mandatory minimum sentence, they're going to serve their term," says Puerini. "Try to figure out how to deal with a guy who is incontinent. If the guy is pooping his pants, the corrections officers say they can't have him in a cell."

As president of the Society of Correctional Physicians, an organization set up to establish high ethical standards in providing health care to those incarcerated, Puerini is arguing to have frail and elderly inmates released from prison: "There has to be the political will to get early compassionate release for elderly and very sick people and I don't see that. We need to push legislators to at least consider it."

Sooner or later, patients like these need to be transferred to an ER for further assessment. When he hears ER doctors and nurses use slang like *incarceritis* and find it amusing, Puerini wonders whether they assume every incarcerated patient is lying for secondary gain.

"That doctor in the emergency room sees the guy in manacles and chains and thinks this guy wants to use him," says Puerini. "He isn't thinking as well as he should about doing real medicine."

This is not just one kind of health-care professional ranting about another. In a document titled *Recognizing the Needs of Incarcerated Patients in the Emergency Department*, the American College of Emergency Physicians had this to say regarding preconceived notions prevalent in the ER: "Many healthcare providers (including nurses, physicians and technicians) view incarcerated patients as unreliable (especially with regard to providing honest personal histories), dangerous and manipulative malingerers."

That, says Puerini, leads ER doctors to send the patient back to prison without diagnosing the problem. "If they're sent back from the emergency room, we may assume they did a thorough assessment and so he must be okay. The next thing you know, the guy dies in his cell."

Puerini knows the risk. He likes to talk about a case that shows just how easily a thing like that can happen.

"The guy's in the segregation unit, and I got called in there to see him," recalls Puerini. "It's a lot harder to see the guys when they're in segregation. They have to come out in manacles and chains. It's a big problem for everybody. We try to put off routine care, because if they're in segregation, it's a big hassle. The prisoner complained of numbness and tingling in his leg. I did a full evaluation and didn't find any objective illness."

Numbness and tingling can be caused by diabetes, a stroke, or a host of other neurological problems. The symptoms can also be faked. Puerini's comment about finding no objective illness is code for saying he found nothing to suggest the segregated prisoner had anything seriously wrong with him.

Puerini decided to wait and see if his patient developed any new symptoms. Four weeks later, the officer in charge of the prisoner asked Puerini to see the prisoner again. In the interim, the prisoner had complained of weakness in the legs. When he began getting a fellow inmate to carry him from his bunk to the toilet, the officer became suspicious.

"He can walk, I know he can walk," the corrections officer said when he asked Puerini to see the prisoner again. "Get this guy to walk to the toilet. He's bullshitting."

Puerini had the prisoner pulled out of segregation and into a room where he could re-examine him. The prisoner couldn't move his legs. He was rushed to hospital.

"The guy had a very aggressive spinal-cord tumour and was dead within six weeks," says Puerini. "I think it's a perfect story because these are the pressures on a physician trying to do correctional medicine. The officer is telling me this guy is bullshit, and I go there and I find very strong evidence for a horrible disease process."

I'm struck by a paradox. As I've shown you, on the outside of the correctional system, most doctors and nurses treat drug seekers with undisguised contempt. Inside the prison wall, doctors like Puerini advocate for the incarcerated felons under their care, and nurses like Nicole Donaldson delight in using humour to get along with hardened criminals with mental health issues.

Dr. Zubin Damania is one doctor on the outside who almost learned the hard way how important it is at least sometimes to check one's suspicions at the door. Damania developed a deep distrust of drug-seeking patients while training as a resident in internal medicine at Stanford University in Stanford, California.

"Working at the County Hospital in Silicon Valley, I was repeatedly dealing with drug seekers and heroin users—to the point that I trusted no one. We would often just say someone was FOS, as in full of shit," says Damania, echoing the slang word SHPOS Bergman first heard in New York City forty years ago.

But sooner or later, everyone gets seriously ill, even drug seekers. "A 30-year-old dude comes in," Damania recalls. "He had a history of heroin and Dilaudid abuse. When I examined him, he complained of pain everywhere. All of the muscles on his face were clenched and he could barely talk.

"I thought he was full of shit. In fact, he had this creepy grin on his face that made me think he was totally effing with us to get Dilaudid. I thought he was a terrible actor. I totally blew him off after telling him I wouldn't give him any narcotics. I even told my intern that he was a classic drug seeker and we shouldn't give in to his nonsense."

Damania gave his assessment to his attending physician, who decided to see the patient for himself. "The attending comes in, takes one look at him and diagnoses tetanus related to the patient's abuse of intravenous drugs."

The grin on the patient's face was a classic sign of tetanus known as *risus sardonicus*, or sardonic smile. It's a clinical term that describes the appearance of the face when the facial muscles are locked into a painful contraction.

Instead of being kicked out of the ER, Damania's patient was intubated and placed on a ventilator in the intensive care unit, where he remained for several weeks. Damania says he thinks about the man often. "He could well have succumbed to complications. I can think of many community hospitals where the doctors would have given the patient narcotics just to get him out of there. That would have been a fatal decision in his case."

You could argue that drug seekers and incarcerated patients are often one and the same. It's health professionals who treat them differently. On the outside, I think, drug seekers make doctors and nurses feel threatened because they remind us that in some doctor-patient relationships, we aren't in control.

Some would say it's the correctional patients' lies that come back to haunt them. Any way you look at it, doctors like Mike Puerini must find the sweet spot between suspicion and trust.

CHAPTER NINE

Harpooning the Whale

On November 24, 2011, the British newspaper the *Daily Mail* reported that Arthur Berkowitz, a 57-year-old passenger on US Airways Flight 901, had to stand for most of the seven hours it took to fly from Anchorage, Alaska, to Philadelphia. The reason? His 400-pound seatmate was so large that when both armrests were raised to accommodate him, the man's bulk spilled over onto Berkowitz's seat.

"He was a real gentleman," Berkowitz told reporters. "The first thing he said to me was: 'I want to apologize—I'm your worst nightmare.'"

Patients as large as the man seated next to Berkowitz are many a doctor's worst nightmare too. Obese and overweight patients represent a plentiful source of new and ongoing business for doctors—and a rather rich source of recent medical slang that is often vicious and pointed. Anesthesiologists have a telling bit of medical argot they use to describe the exercise of inserting an epidural catheter—a flexible tube that's placed through the back into a space in the spinal canal to deliver pain-relief medication—into an obese woman in the late stages of labour. They call it "harpooning the whale."

"I've heard it many times," says Dr. Jay Ross, an anesthesiologist, who is quick to point out he doesn't utter the phrase himself.

The harpoon is the extra-long Tuohy needle used to insert an epidural catheter. A hollow hypodermic needle with a slight curve at the end, the Tuohy was developed to get through the extra layers of tissue in the back. It has to be threaded precisely between the vertebrae in the back. The whale part is self-explanatory.

"You have to get through the skin, the fat and all that," says Ross. "A lot of obese patients have so much fat on their back that you're often struggling to even feel the spinous processes to insert the epidural or the spinal needle in the first place. Sometimes I'll actually ask the patient if it feels like I have placed the needle on the left or the right of the midline."

Increasingly, anesthesiologists use a portable ultrasound machine to locate the epidural space that is the destination of the needle. However, for the many anesthesiologists who don't have one, it's a matter of guesswork. Ross says that with a pregnant woman of average weight, it takes about fifteen minutes to insert an epidural. For obese women, it can take as long as forty-five minutes—even longer. The longer it takes to put in an epidural, the less likely the pain meds will kick in time for the critical stage of labour in which the woman is encouraged to push. Increasingly, Ross and his colleagues warn obese patients up front that there's trouble ahead.

"I used to be very reticent about doing that," says Ross. "I'm a lot less so now because I think there's no real point in beating around the bush. If you don't do it, then they're sort of wondering why you're stabbing their back multiple times for forty-five minutes. It can be very frustrating."

That frustration has turned anesthesiologists into slangmeisters. "The [terms] I'm aware of I try not to use," says Ross. Before he arrived at the hospital where he did his residency, he says, "They used to have an award called the Prince of Whales award. It was awarded to the resident on call who placed obstetrical epidurals in the most tonnage in one shift."

And Ross's hospital wasn't unique. A resident told me there was a Princess of Whales award at the medical school he attended. "It was for the anesthesiologist who put an epidural into the woman with the highest BMI [body mass index]. It was a plaque and it was awarded every year."

Whale isn't the only slang noun used to describe obese patients. And anesthesiology isn't the only hospital domain to boast a flourishing slang directed at obese patients. Dr. Christian Jones recently completed a residency in general surgery in Kansas City. He plans on becoming a trauma surgeon and expects to fix up a lot of obese patients.

"I think in surgery in general—and certainly more and more in trauma over the last ten or fifteen years—there's been a lot of concern about what we euphemistically call 'excessive soft tissue' (a more subtle bit of slang) in the obese patient," says Jones. "I think especially in trauma there are more and more euphemisms being used for that.

"There's *cow*. There's *fluffy*, which is a relatively benign one, I suppose. One that I hadn't heard before I came to the University of Kansas was the *seal sign*. That is when we do an X-ray or CT scan of a patient and find a large amount of soft tissue outside their body cavity. They're just like a seal, with lots of surrounding blubber. The one that I particularly liked, I hate to say, was that on the X-ray it looks like they're a killer whale that just swallowed a seal."

Dr. Mark Ryan, a family doctor in Richmond, Virginia, finished his residency in 2003 and began his career in rural Virginia before moving to Richmond. He's now splitting his time—40 percent teaching and academics, 60 percent patient care. He confirms that surgeons use *fluffy* frequently: "If you're going to do a surgery on somebody and they're obese, the surgery will be a little more difficult because you have to get through the layers of fat tissue before you can get down to the muscle. So the surgeon might describe the patient as being a fluffy person."

Derogatory? You bet. No surgeon would ever refer to a patient as fluffy, a seal or a whale within earshot. Most wouldn't even insinuate it. One resident recalls a time when he and a fellow resident did just that and got busted.

"One of my colleagues referred to a patient as a big fat chick," a resident who trained recently in the U.S. told me. "This was a trauma patient that had come in after a motor vehicle accident. She had relatively minor injuries—some extremity fractures—and no chest, abdominal or pelvic injuries. She didn't have a head injury. Unfortunately, obese patients don't tend to be as injured initially but do have significantly more complications after trauma. And this was a textbook presentation of that.

"She ended up getting a urinary tract infection and a skin ulcer that was very difficult to manage. A new attending trauma surgeon asked, 'Why are all these things happening to her?' My younger, more junior colleague said, 'It's basically because she's a big fat chick.' A couple of us chuckled. There weren't any major laughs or guffaws but there certainly wasn't any admonishment or embarrassment either."

When the resident and the rest of the trauma team entered the patient's room, they were in for a shock. "The patient's father was standing there and he says, 'You know, we can hear you when you're standing outside the door,'" the resident recalls. "He asked us, 'You just call anybody fat without regard to their feelings?'"

The resident says the attending trauma surgeon apologized to the family, but then started to make a bad situation worse: "He said if she weren't overweight, a lot of the complications would not have been happening," he says. "That almost made things more embarrassing for those of us who had been involved."

And the junior resident who called his patient a big fat chick? "I'm fairly certain that colleague hasn't used that term or similar ones since," the resident concludes.

To avoid embarrassing situations like that, surgeons who operate on obese patients have invented argot that can be overheard by patients without being understood.

Jones says one bit of slang that's been making the rounds over the last ten years or so is giving weight a geographic distinction. "You ask a colleague how much a patient weighs. The colleague replies, 'They're one Chicago unit' or 'one Minnesota unit' or 'one Wisconsin unit.' Those are the three most common ones I've heard."

If one Chicago unit means 200 pounds, then a patient who is two Chicago units weighs 400 pounds, a patient who is three Chicago units weighs 600 pounds, and so on. A hospital in Iowa rates obese patients as Iowa 1 to Iowa 4 based on their weight and whether they can fit onto a standard hospital stretcher with both side rails up, one up, or none.

Mark Ryan is also up on the use of geographic slang to identify obese patients. He cares mostly for uninsured patients and those who receive Medicare and Medicaid benefits in Richmond, Virginia, and obesity rates are quite high in his practice. "In Southside Virginia's low-income communities it was a pretty big issue," says Ryan. "An obstetrician-gynecologist would say, 'There's big, and then there's Southside big'—Southside big being heavier and more obese than just obese. It was the sense that people there were heavier than in other parts of the state."

Dr. Marjorie Greenfield of Case Western Reserve University School of Medicine says that at her hospital they used a similar way of saying how much a patient weighs: "Weight was referred to in 'clinic units.' Our clinic is our residents' clinic. The patients who go there are living in poverty and tend to be heavier than the private patients. A clinic unit is about 200 pounds."

Other hospitals across the U.S. use the clinic unit as a way of estimating weights. Greenfield says she hasn't heard about clinic units recently, but that doesn't mean doctors are failing to take note of patients' weight. "People will say her BMI is 60 and maybe roll their eyes," says Greenfield. "But I don't think that that's transmitted to the patients as much as it used to be, and I think it's not as socially acceptable as it used to be."

BMI, or body mass index, is a simple index commonly used to classify weight. It is calculated by dividing a person's weight in kilograms by the square of the person's height in metres. According to the World Health Organization, a BMI of 25 or more is overweight and a BMI of 30 or more is obese.

BMI has also inspired a bit of slang that can easily be spoken in front of patients. "I'm sure you've heard the term *beemer code*," one resident told me. Until he mentioned it, I hadn't. According to the *Urban Dictionary, beemer* is slang for a BMW motorcycle and *bimmer* is argot for a BMW car. I was pretty certain the resident wasn't referring to either. Turns out *beemer* is medical slang for an extra fee doctors can charge to care for an obese patient.

"If you're going to be billing for operating on a patient with morbid obesity, the anesthesiologist will ask the surgeon, or vice-versa, if it is okay to charge a beemer code," says this resident. In a sign of the growing problem of obesity in North America, both Medicaid and some provincial health-care plans have bonus fee codes for patients with a high BMI; these are meant to compensate the anesthesiologist for the extra work caring for morbidly obese patients.

One physician who detests that sort of language is Dr. Arya Sharma. The internationally recognized obesity guru is professor and chair in Obesity Research and Management at the University of Alberta. In 2005, Sharma spearheaded the launch of the Canadian Obesity Network, which has remarkably transformed the landscape of obesity research and management in Canada. He is a fellow of the Council for High Blood Pressure Research of the American Heart Association.

I've got a beached whale in my emergency room—Sharma says he's heard colleagues say this "on a clinical ward where they had a very large patient and everybody thought that was very funny." Sometimes health professionals use gestures and tone of voice instead of words to demonstrate contempt."It's often not just the terminology," Sharma adds. "It's the context in which it's used. It's the acceptance that such terminology finds, and I think it's the state of mind that it puts the provider in that is the problem.

"Very often, it starts with language. If I've got a large woman in distress in front of me, my attitude is going to be very different if I say, 'I've got a whale lying here in my in my exam room and I'm going to have to move the furniture out to make enough space to do a physical examination.'"

Disrespectful language and a disrespectful attitude to the patient—whether it's the tone of the doctor's voice or body language or the time spent at the bedside or listening or talking—affect the quality of care, Sharma says.

The attitude Sharma is talking about is what experts refer to as "weight bias"—the tendency to ascribe negative personality traits to overweight people. Mark Ryan says that "there's still a sense among a certain group of physicians and a certain number of health-care professionals [that maintaining a healthy weight] is a matter of will-power: if you just cared more or tried harder, you wouldn't face this problem. Therefore, it's a personal failure if you're obese."

Dr. Christopher Kinsella, a second-year general surgery resident in St. Louis, Missouri, says he and his colleagues call obese patients slugs. "*Slug* is a huge, huge term for us," says Kinsella, who blogs under the name Topher. "I'm deeply in love with that term. When someone comes in and they're fat and they're clearly lazy, you just know that this person's not going to heal on schedule."

What Kinsella says and what Ryan has observed is backed by studies showing systemic weight bias by health professionals. A study of nearly 2,300 physicians who practise in the United States published in 2012 in the journal *PLOS ONE* demonstrated a strong preference for thin people and both implicit and explicit anti-fat bias. Another study by internist and researcher Dr. Melanie Jay and colleagues published in 2009 in the journal *BMC Health Services Research* concluded that 40 percent of physicians surveyed had a negative reaction toward obese patients. Interestingly, compared to internists, pediatricians were more positively predisposed to obese patients and psychiatrists were less likely to have low expectations of treatment success with overweight patients.

Rebecca Puhl, a clinical psychologist and director of research for the Rudd Center for Food Policy and Obesity at Yale University in New Haven, Connecticut, says physicians ascribe some of the most contemptible patient characteristics to people who are obese. A study of more than 600 doctors found that more than half said obese patients were unattractive, socially awkward and unlikely to take medication as directed. In a review article published in 2001 in the journal *Obesity Research*, Puhl and co-author Kelly Brownell cited research that showed 24 percent of nurses say they are "repulsed" by obese persons.

The weight bias among health professionals is in part a reflection of similar bias in society at large. A study found that two-thirds of Americans are biased against overweight people.

"It's that social acceptability that's it's okay to make fun of fat people because they deserve to be made fun of," says obesity guru Sharma. "It's okay to say obesity is their fault and if they can't be motivated and worried enough to look after themselves, then they really deserve contempt."

It's *overt* contempt that distinguishes how physicians treat obese people compared with other patients. "You would not make a racial slur to a patient," says Sharma. "You would not have a gender thing going on. You would not even dream of doing it. You would be banished from your profession and lose your licence and be kicked out of the hospital because that is completely inappropriate. But when it comes to an obese person, people say, 'Here's the fat guy in room so-and-so.'"

And health professionals don't just make up slang. They spread rumours and make jokes too, says Dr. Simon Field, an ER physician in Halifax. Field was taking a course in the United States when, during a lunch break with a couple of colleagues, the talk turned to massively obese patients and how newer CT scanners were too small to accommodate them safely. "One physician from Texas said his local hospital was sending so many patients to the Houston Zoo to use the zoo's veterinary CT scanner that the zoo complained the humans were jumping the queue on sick and injured animals," Field recalls.

A physician from Florida added that his hospital sent bariatric (obese) patients to Sea World, where the killer whales apparently had their own CT scanner. "Massively obese patients in Orlando ended up in Shamu the killer whale's CT scan machine," Field says the Florida doctor told him.

Sorry, folks, but there's little evidence these alleged transfers actually occur. Here's what a 2007 article in the *Houston Chronicle* had to say: "It's a long-standing urban legend that zoos have jumbo versions of such equipment to help diagnose illnesses in elephants and other huge creatures. But to the disappointment of some doctors, zoo officials must tell them they have no such device."

A story published in the British newspaper *The Telegraph* in January 2012 said National Health Service (NHS) hospitals have resorted to asking zoos and vets to do CT scans on patients who are too obese to fit into hospital scanners. According to the article, Britain's Royal Veterinary College said its CT scanners, "customized for horses, could be used to accommodate patients weighing 30 stone [420 pounds] or more but they would need to get a special licence to scan humans."

But spokespeople for the NHS and the London Zoo both said no such referrals had either taken place or had even been recommended.

An article by *Telegraph* medical correspondent Stephen Adams published in November 2012 said that as an emergency measure, the NHS would rely on scanners usually operated by veterinarians. But, like almost everyone else who has written or spoken about this, the writer was relying on the quotes of sources; I have not seen any articles in which the reporter witnessed obese patients being scanned by a CT designed for large animals.

As for the Shamu scanner, without proof, it's a whale of a tale and probably nothing more.

Legend or true, stories like these prove Sharma's point: even doctors think it's okay to turn obese patients into a punchline.

//////

But if you think doctors' belittling of the obese is simply a case of "weight bias begets a bad attitude," you haven't spent time recently in an operating room caring for patients with morbid obesity—those who are 100 pounds over their ideal weight. Almost without exception, the surgeons, obstetrician-gynecologists and anesthesiologists

I interviewed spoke at length about how difficult it is to care for patients with a BMI north of 40.

"I do think it makes many surgeries much more difficult," says Christian Jones, who can rhyme off a long list of reasons. "The amount of time we have to spend in the operating room is significantly increased by someone who is morbidly or super-obese, compared to someone of normal stature. It is difficult to get a proper look at where we're operating. It is difficult to move things around. Surgery is associated with more and more complications. They have terrible wound-healing problems and very often get wound infections. And patients who are obese tend to have kidney problems, diabetes, skin ulcers and so forth."

When he was doing his residency, Jones recalls, he worked with an attending surgeon who operated frequently on obese patients—not as a bariatric surgeon but as someone who was called on to fix the complications caused by other surgeons. "Since these patients tend to have more complications, very often they need to have repeat surgery," says Jones. "It is quite frustrating."

And it's not just obese adults. Increasingly, surgeons have to operate on morbidly obese adolescents and children.

"I had [an obese] kid who came in with appendicitis that was ruptured," says a resident who is training in the Midwestern U.S. When that happens, the usual plan is to admit the patient to hospital for several days of intravenous antibiotics to treat the inflamed appendix and the infection that has spread through the abdominal cavity. Then, once the inflammation has settled down, the patient is discharged from hospital for several more weeks of antibiotics until surgeons deem it safe to remove the appendix. Thin patients usually require three or four days in hospital. His obese adolescent patient was hospitalized much longer than that.

"This kid was here for a record two weeks," says the resident. "This was a kid who was just *very* overweight, a kid who I think has physiologically deranged her body. It took two weeks for this kid to get to the point where she could evacuate her bowels, have her pain controlled with pills, and walk. There's no good reason for that."

After all of that, the resident says, the teenager will still have to return to hospital to have her appendix removed—a prospect he was dreading: "She's not going to recover from surgery on schedule. She's not going be an active participant in her own recovery at all."

Here is what another resident said to me when I told him that story: "You hate that person as a patient. You operate on them because you have to."

The sense I've gotten from talking to surgical residents is that they didn't sign up to operate on bariatric patients. They look with envy at mentors who are a lot closer to the end of their careers and won't have to spend too many years operating on large patients.

If it makes them feel better, it's not just residents who are doing the complaining; so are experienced attending physicians, including Dr. Marcus Burnstein, a colorectal surgeon. "I don't think the lay public knows how much of a risk factor obesity is for abdominal operations. Non-surgeons may not fully appreciate it either. Getting in and out of the abdomen for open or minimally invasive cases, exposing the operative field, handling the tissues—everything is much more difficult. And patients have a tougher time in the post-op period.

"You have to fight the urge to get angry at the patient for being so fat that the usually simple task of exteriorizing a segment of bowel [creating a hole, or ostomy, on the abdomen so that bowel movements go into a bag attached to the abdomen] has been turned into a nightmare."

The more Burnstein talks about operating on obese patients, the more frustrated he becomes. "It is also physically much more demanding on the whole team to operate on obese patients. Holding retractors to help with exposure can become exhausting. And if there is a huge pannus, the weight of the apron of the fatty abdominal wall can put stress on the abdominal wound and on the stoma [the opening where the bag is attached] and create healing problems."

A pannus—also called an abdominal apron—is a flap of excess skin, fat and tissue at the bottom of the abdomen. It occurs in overweight and morbidly obese patients as well as on people who have lost large amounts of weight and have excess skin. Obese patients can have difficulty moving around because the pannus hangs down over their knees or between their legs. A bulging pannus can make it difficult to tie shoelaces and even to see one's feet. It makes it difficult to bathe properly and therefore to remove offensive body odour. It's also a frequent cause of back pain.

Those are some of the obese patient's problems. When it comes time to do an emergency Caesarean section, the excess weight becomes the obstetrician's problem.

Surgeons who have to deal with a pannus have given it some unflattering nicknames. In the U.S. Midwest and in Boston, it's called the "Milwaukee goiter." In the southern United States, they call it a "Bojangleoma," a nifty bit of slang. The suffix –oma means "tumour." Bojangle comes from Bojangles' Famous Chicken 'n Biscuits, a restaurant chain in the American South.

Whatever you call it, a pannus is bad news for the surgeon or resident who has to cut through it in order to operate underneath it.

"You're digging into a hole with the edges falling in," says a former OBGYN resident who switched careers to become a GP. "You can't fortify the edges of the hole or the pit—horrible to say. You can't see as well. You need special equipment for the physicians to get high enough to be able to dig deep enough into the belly to get the baby out. I'm a tall person and I remember once being up on a riser and having to be in the belly up almost my shoulder trying to feel for the baby."

It's also a lot of extra work—for more than one person.

"You need at least two extra people, i.e., four more hands, to retract a pannus," says the former obstetrics resident. "The junior resident and the medical student would be the pannus holders. To hold it is a sign of being the lowest on the food chain. It's super slippery and it's usually pretty smelly. It's shameful that we as a profession would feel a little degraded by holding the pannus."

Dr. Marjorie Greenfield, the OBGYN at Case Western University School of Medicine, says Caesarean sections are physically demanding operations when the woman is morbidly obese. Greenfield wouldn't dream of using derogatory slang to describe obese patients. But she—like everyone else I interviewed—recites chapter and verse on the extreme challenges of caring for large patients in her line of work.

"You have to hold the pannus up," she says. "This is sort of horrifying, but what we actually do is put tape on the pannus and tape it up to the anesthesia screen as we're setting up for the Caesarean so that we can get to the lower abdomen.

"I can only imagine what that seems like to the patient—to have her big fat stomach taped up to the surgical drape with pieces of adhesive tape to try to get to where you're making your incision. Otherwise, what you end up doing is holding the pannus up with one arm while you're trying to do everything with your other arm. It's very hard on your body as you're going through the surgery."

And after all that effort to get the baby out, the challenges for mom and for the surgeons looking after her don't end. Obese women who have Caesareans are at huge risk for infections, says the OBGYN resident. "You know that when you cut into their skin that you're going to see them in the emergency room four or six weeks later with a soft-tissue infection. It's challenging, at best."

In general, a C-section is performed when a vaginal delivery would put the health of the baby or the mother at risk. According to a review article published in 2012 in the *North American Journal of Medical Sciences*, obesity has a dramatic effect on the outcome of the pregnancy. It increases the risk of gestational diabetes, high blood pressure, pre-eclampsia (high blood pressure and significant amounts of protein in the urine that can lead to a life-threatening condition), pre-term delivery, blood clots in the lung and other conditions. There are increased risks for the baby as well. Morbid obesity itself significantly increases the likelihood of a C-section delivery. In a study published in the journal *Anesthesiology* in 1993, the rate of emergency C-section was just 9 percent in women of normal weight and up to 50 percent in women who are morbidly obese.

The female OBGYN resident I spoke to said it can be quite difficult to tell whether an obese woman requires an emergency C-section or can be delivered vaginally. "We talk about vaginal pannus and vulvar pannus and the labial pannus," says a former OBGYN resident. "There's just more of all that tissue and it's really hard to find the cervix often. You need an extra large speculum. You can't position them on the bed."

These aren't theoretical concerns. I heard a story from an attending OBGYN that made my heart stop.

The doctor was doing a vaginal delivery on a very obese woman. The first part of the delivery took place without incident. Suddenly, a fetal monitor attached by the doctors to make sure things were okay showed that the baby's heart rate was slowing down—a sign that the baby was in distress. With each passing second, there was a greater and greater risk that the baby would asphyxiate and suffer permanent brain damage. To make it as easy as possible for the baby's head to pass through the birth canal, the OBGYN did a large episiotomy.

An episiotomy is a surgical incision made in the perineum, the skin and underlying tissue roughly between the vagina and the anus. It's done during the last stages of labour and delivery to expand the opening of the vagina to prevent tearing. Once commonplace, episiotomies are performed as little as possible today, in preference to a more natural childbirth in which a tear may or may not occur spontaneously.

The woman was so large that the OBGYN couldn't make out the anatomical landmarks to do a proper episiotomy. She made the incision as quickly as possible and got the baby out safely.

Crisis over, the obstetrician prepared to stitch the episiotomy—or so she thought. As she pulled back the skin billowing voluminously on both sides of the woman's vulva and perineum, the OBGYN was astounded to see that both were completely intact. The doctor went looking for the incision she knew she had made, and realized with a gasp that she had made it through the woman's thigh, which she had mistaken for the vulva.

It was only then that the OBGYN realized that at the time the baby was in distress, it had already been born, but was suffocating under the mother's large thigh.

Stories like these get passed around by everyone from attending physicians to residents, along with the inevitable black humour, such as having to find a veterinary speculum—or one large enough to push away the floppy vaginal tissue. These jokes—distasteful though they may be—come from frustration mixed with despair.

"You get lots more skin and vulvar infections," says the former OBGYN resident. "I'm ashamed to say but it's smellier. I would always feel ashamed of myself that I'm frustrated about this. I don't want to do it because I'm thinking how much harder it is for her. No matter how hard I'm trying to hide my feelings, she must have radar for them. How humiliating must that be for her that I'm frustrated doing the vaginal exam?"

Arya Sharma agrees that it's paramount for health professionals to empathize with bariatric patients. "When you actually think of a woman lying there in labour, that's probably one of the most vulnerable moments that you can imagine anybody to be in," says Sharma. "She is surrounded by doctors and nurses who are using this kind of language. Irrespective of whether she hears the language or not, from a professional standpoint it's an ethical question."

But to many health professionals, it's also a clinical question. In the OR, on the other side of the surgical drapes, anesthesiologists like Dr. Jay Ross have their own troubles keeping morbidly obese patients alive during surgery. Being obese means that the tissue inside the throat and the airway is also large and floppy. "That makes getting the endotracheal tube into the trachea more difficult and even ventilating them more difficult because it's sometimes harder to get a seal of the ventilation mask over the mouth," says Ross.

Ross says these problems mean that the oxygen levels of obese patients can drop quickly. These patients are more likely than thinner patients to die on the table.

I put to Dr. Sharma the litany of clinical issues related to the treatment of morbidly obese patients that I heard from dozens of attending surgeons, OBGYNs, anesthesiologists and residents.

"Well, it's all true," Sharma concedes. "What makes it different is the attitude with which you approach it. We can have difficult patients who present us with a technical challenge or a diagnostic challenge. You need to be professionally trained to know how to address it. You need to make sure you have the right equipment in place that is going to allow you to deliver the best care.

"When it comes to obese people, we often don't have that equipment. You're looking for seven guys to help get this guy out of his bed and on a commode when a ceiling lift can be operated by one person and can do this in a much safer way, both for the provider and for the patient. But if you don't have the ceiling lift, you're lacking the equipment that's out there. It's available."

Lifting a morbidly obese patient is no minor issue. Generally speaking, patients can transfer themselves from a stretcher to the operating room table because they're awake. Immediately following surgery, when they're just beginning to awaken from anesthesia, they are usually unable to transfer themselves back to the stretcher.

"I know of a resident who actually slipped a disc lifting a patient from the bed to the gurney," says Ross. "She had to have an operation after that. So there are obvious health risks to us as well, like throwing out your back and straining muscles. You're obviously also concerned whether you can actually get these patients safely from one bed to another without hurting them or having them fall on the floor."

Even that example didn't move Sharma.

"That resident had no business even trying to lift that patient," he says, "because that resident should have known that she was putting herself at risk trying to do that—unless this was a huge emergency and there was absolutely no other option. If I'm putting myself at risk as a provider, that is unprofessional conduct. We're talking 2013 here; we have lifting devices. We've got equipment and materials that have been specifically designed for use in larger patients."

When I asked Jay Ross about using a mechanized lift in the OR for heavier patients, he called it "not a bad idea," as though no one at his hospital had thought of getting one.

Bariatric equipment exists but it isn't cheap. For example, in 2011, a blog written by Whitecoat published on kevinmd.com notes that Boston Emergency Medical Services had recently debuted an ambulance with a mini-crane and reinforced stretcher to transport patients weighing up to 850 pounds—at a cost of tens of thousands of dollars per ambulance. That prompted Whitecoat to ask this question: "Should it ever be right to tell patients that if they let themselves get so obese that traditional ambulances can't carry them that dispatchers will refuse transport and they will be responsible for their own transportation to the hospital?"

When a doctor doesn't know how to care for bariatric patients, Sharma says, it's the doctor's fault; when the doctor can't care properly for these patients because the hospital or ambulance service don't purchase bariatric equipment, it's the system's fault. Either way, doctors are becoming increasingly frustrated, and bariatric patients are losing their dignity—and all too often something more.

In 2012, Ida Davidson of Shrewsbury, Massachusetts, went looking for a new primary-care physician. According to a story posted to wcvb.com in August 2012, Davidson called on Dr. Helen Carter, who refused to take her on because at the time Davidson weighed more than 200 pounds. "After three consecutive injuries [with other patients] trying to care for people over 250 pounds, my office is unable to accommodate a certain weight and we put a limit on it," Carter told reporter Pam Cross.

In 2011, the *South Florida Sun Sentinel* reported that fifteen of 105 obstetrics and gynecology practices likewise refused to see otherwise healthy women who weighed more than 200 pounds. A 2013 article in the *New England Journal of Medicine*, bioethicist Holly Fernandez Lynch noted that Ethical Rule 10.05 of the American Medical Association (AMA) permits doctors to refuse to treat patients whose medical problems are beyond their competence and to provide services that go against the doctor's personal, moral or religious beliefs. The AMA adds that doctors cannot refuse to care for patients based on race, gender, sexual orientation, gender identity "or any other criteria that would constitute invidious discrimination."

Fernandez Lynch wrote that the right of doctors to refuse to care for patients has been reduced further by state laws that prohibit what are known as places of "public accommodation" (including doctors' offices and hospitals) from discriminating—not just on the basis of the AMA criteria, but also on "medical condition, disability or other personal features." The Americans with Disabilities Act (ADA) of 1990 prohibits discrimination "in any place of public accommodation."

Does that mean doctors cannot refuse to care for bariatric patients? Not necessarily. Fernandez Lynch goes on to say that refusing patients based on the ADA might be perfectly legal if it can be shown that an obese person is not disabled: "Discrimination on some grounds may be legally impermissible, whereas discrimination on other grounds is only morally blameworthy, but these cases are newsworthy precisely because they are so unexpected from a profession with a strong tradition of helping people in need and rejecting the stigmas that may bias other members of society."

Dr. David Katz, one of America's most celebrated experts in obesity, notes that obese patients are less likely than thin patients to receive appropriate care of medical problems that have little if anything to do with their weight. "I met a woman who should have had cancer screening tests but had not," Katz wrote in 2011 in the *Huffington Post*. "I met a woman who should have had screening tests for cardiac risk and [who should have] received select immunizations—who had not. I met a woman who had been driven from any and all benefits that modern medicine might offer her by the cold and denigrating judgment offered her by almost every modern medical practitioner she had met."

Dr. Marjorie Greenfield believes that obese patients need to accept that, in some cases, circumstances may compromise their care. "I don't think it's on purpose, but I think a lot of times people can't get the same level of care because there's a part of the quality of your care that has to do with your participation," says Greenfield. "There's sort of a price that you pay in terms of the quality of care you can get either when you're very obese or also when you haven't gotten good prenatal care and haven't taken good care of yourself. And I think there's a price that you pay in terms of outcomes for the pregnancy—like the rate of birth defects, labour progress not going well, things that are actual complications of pregnancy."

To Dr. Arya Sharma, that's blaming patients for being the way they are. "Let's assume that you're working in a rehabilitation centre where part of your job is dealing with paraplegic patients and getting upset at these paraplegic guys who are peeing in their pants all the time," says Sharma. "If that's your attitude, you shouldn't be working in a place that looks after people who have paraplegic problems."

Sharma says if you take "paraplegic" and substitute "bariatric," it's exactly the same problem. The Centers for Disease Control says that 68.8 percent of Americans are either overweight or obese. Close to four million Americans weigh more than 300 pounds, and close to half a million (mostly men) weigh more than 400 pounds.

"You should have known that two-thirds of your patients are going to be overweight or obese," says Sharma. "If you don't like overweight and obese people, then you shouldn't be in medical practice—period."

Far from shaming patients into slimming down, there's evidence that the bias against obese people has the opposite effect. A 2013 study of more than 6,000 people published in the journal *PLOS ONE* found that people who experienced weight discrimination are more than twice as likely to remain obese as those who do not experience such prejudice.

Sharma says it's not too late to turn things around. "Everybody went into medical school because they wanted to help people who have problems, and being obese is a problem," he says. "And even if I don't have a treatment and I don't know what the hell I'm talking about, at least I can show concern and understanding and empathy, and say that I cannot possibly imagine what it is like waking up every morning and being 300 pounds and then realizing that you're going to have to lift those 300 pounds out of your bed, shower, clean yourself and dress."

There are uncomfortable parallels between the slang used by doctors to talk about obese patients today and the slang term GOMER, popularized by Dr. Stephen Bergman in *The House of God.* "These are the new GOMERs," says Bergman. "The GOMER still exists but care of those people has actually improved a great deal in terms of medical care and hospice care and other kinds of care for the elderly. They've made big strides."

And obese patients? "I think the epidemic is like a tsunami coming at us," says Bergman. "I can't imagine being a surgeon operating on these people. Imagine if you had to do that surgery all the time."

For those who do it, no imagination is required.

CHAPTER TEN

Frequent Flyers

A woman enters the ER where Not Nurse Ratched is on duty. By the time she arrives at the registration desk, her name, birth date and allergies—even her social security number—have already been typed into the computer. A game of rock-paper-scissors has determined which triage nurse has to take the patient this time.

I'll call the patient Anna. She's in her early forties, weighs close to 400 pounds and has missing teeth. Her multiple tattoos are visible because she's inappropriately dressed for the weather. She's been known, for example, to walk into the ER in the dead of winter with bare feet and wearing nothing but a tank top and sweatpants. Her clothes are often unwashed and her body carries a stale smell.

Anna is familiar to the ER staff at this Kansas community hospital because she visits several times a week. Not Nurse Ratched knows Anna well. Too well. After being triaged by the rock-paper-scissors loser, Anna is placed in her section of the emergency department.

It's a busy night. Not Nurse Ratched is already caring for two patients—one with a serious illness, the other suffering a trauma—

when she gets to Anna. Thankfully, assessing Anna usually doesn't take much time: the ER nurse is familiar with her medical history, and Anna knows the routine.

"Hi, Anna," Not Nurse Ratched says. "What is it tonight?"

Anna never takes offence at the nurse's direct line of questioning. In fact, she appreciates the ER nurse's efficiency. "Abdominal pain. I can't stop puking."

"What's your pain?" Not Nurse Ratched asks, referring to a standard scale used in the ER to assess pain, though it varies depending on who's asking. I usually ask patients to name the most pain they've ever been in, label that a 10, and then rate their current discomfort by comparison. On a scale concocted by Not Nurse Ratched, childbirth is an 8.

"A 10," Anna answers.

"Right," says the ER nurse matter-of-factly. Anna's pain is always a 10.

After checking Anna's vital signs and her oxygen saturation, Not Nurse Ratched determines Anna's not, in fact, sick. Later, the ER physician on duty does a history and physical examination and comes to the same conclusion. But given how busy the ER is that night, no one's available to discharge Anna right away, so she has to wait. Anna doesn't mind. She props herself up in bed, turns on the TV and cracks a can of soda she's brought with her.

Regardless of her apparent comfort, Anna repeatedly rings the call bell, complaining of nausea and requesting an IV with pain medication. Not Nurse Ratched keeps sticking her head back in the room, repeating the same thing each time: "You're not getting an IV. You're waiting for me to discharge you."

When, even after these repeated statements, the call bell rings yet again, Not Nurse Ratched begins to lose her patience. She marches into Anna's room to tell her one last time there is no way she is getting an IV. Anna listens calmly, sticks her fingers down her throat, and vomits on the nurse's leg.

///////

Anna is what ER doctors and nurses call a *frequent flyer*, someone who visits the hospital over and over again. A term known to health professional and laypeople alike, it's borrowed from the loyalty programs offered by many airlines. Irony underlies its medical use. In the airline industry, the loyalty of the frequent flyer is wanted; in medicine, we would just as soon have our repeat customers take their loyalty to some other hospital.

Frequent flyer is a polite way to refer to patients I call avid consumers of health services. Medical lexicon is replete with far more denigrating synonyms. Some of the doctors and nurses I interviewed for this book call them cockroaches.

In a 1993 article titled "Medical Slang and Its Functions," published in the journal *Social Science & Medicine*, Robert Coombs and his co-authors wrote that the slang name *crock*—as in "crock of shit"—is used for "a patient with no ascertainable, measurable physical problem—often a patient with a psychiatric disorder."

Coombs and his co-authors also uncovered the terms *groupie*, defined as a patient "who repeatedly comes to the Emergency Room without a real emergency," and *curly toe*, which refers to "an old bum with toenails so long they curl over"—a common condition of homeless people, who are among the most common frequent flyers.

The medical penchant for using acronyms shows up once again in conversations about frequent flyers. In the compilation by Coombs and his colleagues, CLL—which in real medicine stands for chronic lymphocytic leukemia—is short for "chronic low-life." The acronym NPTG is the abbreviated version of "no place to go."

If you're getting the impression frequent flyers aren't exactly liked by health professionals, you're right. There are many reasons for this. For one thing, a large percentage of frequent flyers in the U.S. are too poor to pay their bills.

But lack of money or reimbursable health care are not the only reasons. Even those who are eligible to receive full health care coverage may fail to do the necessary paperwork to maintain their coverage. Or they have no fixed address and therefore fail the residency test necessary to obtain a health card or a driver's licence. I call these sorts of patients anti-system people, because they've simply dropped off the map.

Coombs et al. documented the use of *nonpayoma* and *negative wallet biopsy* when patients can't pay their hospital bills and the financial hit has to be absorbed by the hospital. The nursing magazine *Scrubs* says the term *negative wallet biopsy* is invoked in the U.S. "when a patient is transferred to a cheaper, less intensive hospital after discovering he has no health insurance."

But money isn't the only reason health professionals view frequent flyers with contempt. To many of them, frequent flyers look and act as if they have no interest in improving their health. Like Anna, they are often obese. They have uncontrolled high blood pressure, as well as uncontrolled diabetes and elevated cholesterol. Often, they're heavy smokers. They seem to have little insight into the connection between their bad lifestyle habits and their health. They tend to be passive participants in their own wellness. They often offer very little useful information as to why they have come to the hospital. Though they visit the ER often, they seem to have little or no interest in taking steps to reduce the frequency of their visits.

I can remember a frequent flyer I'll call Donald, now deceased. When I used to see him, Donald was in his late sixties and would come in every five to seven days complaining of chest tightness. Donald had fibromyalgia, a muscular condition that can sometimes cause chest pain that mimics a heart attack. He used to take acetaminophen to relieve the pain. A short, heavyset man with white hair and broad cheekbones, Donald would walk into the ER clutching his chest.

Of limited intelligence, Donald often gave one-word answers to my questions. If I asked what was wrong with him, he would answer "pain" and fire back the question, "Is it the fibro?" I would order an electrocardiogram and blood tests to rule out a heart attack, both of which would invariably be normal. When I visited Donald's bedside later to give him the good news, he would invariably ask: "Can I go now?" as if—irrespective of the tests—he had decided it was simply time to leave. I must have gone through this ritual with Donald 100 times over a fifteen-year period. That doesn't include the many times he saw my colleagues.

A variant of the frequent flyer is the parent who repeatedly brings a child to the ER for what nurses and doctors believe are trivial reasons. Call that phenomenon "frequent flyer by proxy." In Chapter 4, a pediatric ER physician talked about parents who bring their children to the ER for the same problem again and again without any evidence that they've followed through on the advice given on previous visits: "When there's maybe a psychosocial element to the presentation of the child, a parent could probably be doing a better job raising their kid. That's a nice way of saying it."

Psychosocial is another code word health professionals use frequently. They use it to indicate there's nothing seriously wrong with the patient—at least not anything that the doctor has been trained to fix. When a patient—with or without a parent—bounces back like a boomerang, health professionals feel like they're doing something wrong and they get frustrated.

Physicians and nurses often put hours of effort into taking histories, doing physical examinations, ordering tests and providing intensive nursing care to frequent flyers—for no apparent long-term benefit. At other times, we feel as if we've gotten to know the frequent flyer so well that we stop doing any sort of a workup at all. Often, we busy ourselves fixing minor problems the patient has—fluids for dehydration, sandwiches for hunger and Valium to help the patient dry out from an alcohol binge—without getting at the root cause for the visit. *Treat 'em and street 'em* is the slang term for this type of care.

Something is wrong with a system in which patients come back to the ER again and again and again with the same problem. On both sides of the border, the North American health-care system does little to encourage patients to seek care outside the ER or, in many cases, provides them with few alternatives.

The number of visits per frequent flyer is jaw-dropping. Not Nurse Ratched's patient Anna is approaching her five-hundredth ER visit over several years. In 2013, the *Louisville Courier-Journal* reported that Dennis Manners—who suffers from alcoholism and seizures—visited the ER at University Hospital in Louisville 337 times in less than two years, racking up $626,143 in charges he couldn't pay.

One doctor trying to do something about frequent flyers is Jeffrey Brenner, a primary-care physician in Camden, New Jersey. Brenner is the founder and executive director of the Camden Coalition of Healthcare Providers, a group that works with allied health professionals and hospitals to improve health care for Camden's 78,000 residents.

"In Camden, we found a patient who'd been to the ER 113 times in one year," said Brenner. "We found a patient up in Trenton, New Jersey, who'd been 450 times in a year."

Compared with the entire population, these examples are extreme. The Centers for Disease Control reported that in 2011, the U.S. had 136.1 million visits to emergency departments out of a population of nearly 314 million—approaching just one visit for every two people per year.

Frequent flyers are disproportionate ER users because the ER is the one place that can't turn them away, thanks to federal laws. Kentucky, where Dennis Manners lives, has a very high rate of ER visits—549 for every 1,000 people, compared with the U.S. national average of 428 (as reported by the Centers for Disease Control). Across the U.S., the number per 1,000 people ranges from a relatively paltry 266 in Hawaii to a whopping 736 in the District of Columbia.

If frequently flyers are in the wrong place, Jeffrey Brenner is trying to do something about it. He coined *superutilizer* as a less pejorative term for patients who flock to the ERs of Camden, where for ten years he's been studying billing data from all three hospitals that serve the city. "They're often in the ER because the health-care system doesn't do a good job of taking care of them," he says.

And Brenner also discovered that superutilizers are not just an ER problem. He found that just 1 percent of patients in one part of Camden are responsible for 30 percent of all of the city's health-care costs (of which ER costs are only a fraction), and 20 percent are responsible for 90 percent of the total. Brenner found that in some cases, extraordinarily high rates of health-care consumption can be traced not just to Camden districts but to city blocks, right down to individual apartment buildings.

Brenner calls these places "medical hotspots." And they aren't confined to Camden. They can be found all over the United States and Canada. The west side of Saskatoon is another medical hotspot. Known by local experts as one of Saskatoon's core neighbourhoods, the west side has the highest rate of new HIV infections in Canada, and higher-than-average rates of diabetes, depression, addiction, sexually transmitted diseases and hepatitis C. Its infant mortality rate is higher than in war-torn Bosnia. Like their counterparts in Camden, local residents visit the emergency room at St. Paul's Hospital, which is the heart of the west side, as a means of getting basic health care—not just once or twice, but many more times, making them superutilizers in Brenner's book.

Stephen Lewis, a health policy analyst in Saskatoon, has been documenting the problems in the town's core neighbourhoods for years. He says poverty leads to lack of things that well-off people take for granted—a safe place to live, nourishing food, immunizations, education and access to good primary medical care. Patients who lack these end up sicker, more injured and older before their time. In other words, they morph into superutilizers who frequent the ER at St. Paul's Hospital.

"St. Paul's Hospital is essentially their primary-care centre," says Lewis. "There are large numbers of people who get what they need by going that route." He says the people who live in the area suffer high rates of injury and "there are also higher-than-usual rates of admission for pneumonia and conditions like that because of poor housing, poor lifestyles and so on."

Just a block away from St. Paul's Hospital, I met up with Dr. Ryan Meili, a family doctor who knows these patients all too well. Meili works at Westside Community Clinic in Saskatoon's core community of Riversdale.

"The majority of our patients are First Nations or Métis," says Meili. "We do have a number of refugee or immigrant patients as well. We've seen a great explosion in HIV and hepatitis C as a result of a big increase in substance abuse in the neighbourhood. The patients we see are really the folks who live here and are struggling with those issues."

Back in Camden, one of the most important discoveries to come from Brenner's research is that not all frequent flyers are the uninsured poor. "My work isn't poverty work," he says. "I happen to be working in the poorest city in America, but my work is really about health-care redesign for patients who are very complex and sick."

And you don't even have to be poor to be a frequent flyer, says Brenner. "Even in a wealthy community, as you get older, more frail and disabled, you collect into specific kinds of buildings. I think the challenge for the problem is that [superutilizers are] a very diverse group, a very heterogeneous group," says Brenner. "If I said to you that all high utilizers are homeless, I'd be wrong. It's only a subset of them. If I said to you that all drug addicts are high utilizers, I'd be wrong.

"If you're blind, if you're deaf, if you're disabled, if you're in a wheelchair, if you don't speak English, if you're illiterate, if you're developmentally delayed, if you're depressed, if you're overwhelmed, if you're just older, if you've got complex co-morbidities (more than one of diabetes, chronic kidney disease, cancer, etc.), if you don't have family support, if you're poor—the whole system starts breaking down."

Brenner reminds me of a frequent flyer I'll call Sarah. When I first met Sarah, she was a 21-year-old with chronic depression related to borderline personality disorder. She used to come to the ER after cutting her wrists or taking an overdose of Tylenol. To remove the Tylenol from Sarah's intestines, we would have her swallow a nausea-inducing thick black sludge of activated charcoal mixed with sorbitol. If she was found to have toxic levels of Tylenol in her bloodstream, we would have to give her an antidote called n-acetylcysteine or Mucomyst.

When Sarah came to the ER in an agitated state, I would give her an injection of haloperidol and Lorazepam to calm her down. If she was intoxicated, I would give her thiamine because up to 15 percent of intoxicated patients have low thiamine levels. If, after taking care of her non-psychiatric needs, Sarah said she still felt suicidal, I'd refer her to a psychiatric hospital. Almost invariably, the doctors there would decline to admit her because she didn't meet well-established clinical criteria for admission.

I must have gone through that ritual fifty or more times over a fifteen-year period. Though what I did sounds complicated, it's really an elaborate version of treat 'em and street 'em—since nothing I ever did got at the root causes of why Sarah kept coming back to the ER.

As Sarah got older, she developed severe high blood pressure. Her doctor put her on a complex regime of blood pressure pills. In time, she started coming to the ER with fainting episodes that were due to overdosing on the blood pressure medications. On several occasions, she had to be admitted to the intensive care unit. They'd patch her up and send her back to the street, only to see her return.

It's tempting to chalk up Sarah's frequent-flyer status to her psychiatric history. But as she got older, her cumulative medical problems were no different from those of almost any elderly patient I see frequently in the ER.

Frequent flyers become complex for myriad reasons. They might be elderly or cognitively impaired. They might have multiple medical problems or difficulty staying mobile. They might be homeless or have substance abuse. Often, they have mental health problems that make many ER doctors and nurses wish they'd take their business elsewhere.

"Many of us will end up in that position later in our life in which our health fails," says Brenner. "The system becomes incredibly confusing and difficult to use. So what I don't want to do is stereotype them and say all superutilizers are one type of patient. If it were that easy, we would've fixed the problem a long time ago."

There's no doubt that the North American model of doctor remuneration encourages frequent flyers. The U.S. has a mixture of private and publicly funded health care, while Canada has a single-payer publicly funded system. Despite the differences, physicians in both countries are paid based largely on volume. "Even in the emergency room," says Brenner, "you make more money treating head colds than you do treating really sick people."

Despite big differences in their respective health-care systems, doctors in both the U.S. and Canada don't get paid enough to spend time unpacking the complex problems of frequent flyers. In both countries, they are able make more money treating easier problems because they take far less time—which means they see far more patients per hour.

It's no accident that in Camden, the top four reasons people visit the ER are head colds, viral infections, sore throats and earaches; together, Brenner says, these four minor ailments account for 12,000 ER visits every year in the New Jersey city.

///////

Although frequent flyer usually refers to a patient who comes to the ER, the term can also be used to talk about patients who frequent offices and clinics. Dr. Grumpy, the American neurologist blogger, says the frequent flyers he sees (he calls them cockroaches) tend to suffer from chronic pain. Chronic pain syndromes, such as persistent migraines and fibromyalgia, are both difficult to diagnose and difficult to treat. Patients suffering from these ailments often return to the doctor's office despite the physician's inability to help them.

Paradoxically, the cockroaches Dr. Grumpy writes about are tidy and well mannered. "I think it's their persistent nature that earned them the name cockroach," Dr. Grumpy says. "You just can't get rid of them. They just keep coming back."

One of these patients is a woman who started seeing Dr. Grumpy in her mid-thirties. She complained of chronic headaches and neck pain. Dr. Grumpy ran multiple tests and tried the patient on nearly twenty different medications. When none worked, Dr. Grumpy started to run out of ideas. "I had suggested multiple times she see a specialist at a university nearby, because I really had nothing else to offer her," he says. "And yet she refused to go."

Now, about eight years after her first visit, the appointments follow a repetitive script. Dr. Grumpy begins by asking, "How are you?" The patient responds by describing the same list of symptoms she describes every visit. Dr. Grumpy reviews her medications and re-examines the tests. Then, as he does every appointment, he suggests she see a neurologist and notes she need not come back since there's nothing else he can do to help her. "Then the patient walks right out front and makes a follow-up appointment with my secretary," Dr. Grumpy says.

"There's just never any resolution. It just goes on and on until either they give up or you retire or they die, or the doctor dies."

Dr. Grumpy wonders if coming to his office fills some sort of need for the frequent flyers he sees. "I can only assume there's some sort of psychological dependency. Maybe coming to the doctor is her whole life." He notes that cockroaches tend to schedule their appointments "three years in advance and be there ten minutes early."

ER nurse Not Nurse Ratched believes that although her frequent flyer patient Anna complains of chest or abdominal pain, the real reason for her visits to the ER is anxiety. "For some reason, she gets some kind of need met from being at the emergency department." Once, the ER nurse overheard a doctor talking to Anna about the underlying reason for her visits. "I think that your issue is psychological," the doctor said, "and I think that by feeding into it I'm only making you sicker."

Not Nurse Ratched thinks the doctor had a point. "Our responsibil-ity is to the patient's well-being," she says. "It is not to her well-being if you continue to just treat her and roll your eyes at her. We're making her sick by all this radiation and testing that she doesn't need."

Unfortunately, even if the ER staff were to acknowledge Anna's psychological problems, she would never be accepted for admission to a psychiatric hospital. I found it was often the same with Sarah. A patient's illness has to be considered by a psychiatrist or a psychiatric resident as far more severe than anxiety—think suicide or psychotic break—in order to qualify for admission to a psychiatric facility.

Knowing on some level that she has nowhere else to go, Anna goes to great lengths to manipulate her symptoms in order to stay in the ER, including making herself vomit to the point of getting dehydrated and even having a rapid heartbeat.

Anna reminds me of Donald, my serial patient with chest pain. Donald was a lonely widower. In his most lucid moments in the ER, he would speak of how much he missed his wife. The subject would frequently bring tears to his eyes. Still, no matter how many times I tried to help him see a connection between his sadness and his chest pain, he still kept coming back complaining of physical symptoms.

Whether they visit the ER where I work in Toronto, or one in Camden, the fundamental reason frequent flyers see us is that they can't get the care they need someplace more suitable. Dr. Jeffrey Brenner says this points to a lack of primary care, the kind of medicine usually served up by family doctors, internists and nurse practitioners.

What Brenner is talking about is increasingly referred to as the medical home, sometimes referred to as a patient-centred medical home. It's a team-based model of health-care delivery that provides continuous and comprehensive health care to patients with the goal of keeping them healthy and as far away from a hospital as possible. The leader of the team can be a physician, nurse practitioner or physician assistant.

Brenner says he thinks our health-care system reflects our values as a society. "I think that in the last fifty years, we got very wooed by major advances in medicine. When we turn on the TV and see hearts being transplanted, Siamese twins being separated, you know it's almost magical."

These apparent medical miracles created the sense that doctors can and will do anything to save a life. As the professionals acquired more knowledge and medical prowess, non-medical people came to feel inadequate to handle even minor illnesses and injuries themselves. No wonder people just go to the ER instead of trying to fix a problem themselves.

You don't have to be a patient or a physician in North America to understand what Brenner is talking about. America is dealing with a chronic shortage of family doctors. Recently, the *Annals of Family Medicine* estimated that there are 210,000 primary care physicians in active practice, and the percentage of American physicians who do primary care has been shrinking. To meet the needs of the population, by 2025, the nation will require an additional 52,000.

The solution, says Brenner, is to provide frequent flyers with the care that's missing. For Brenner, the first step was to take the health-care utilization data he gleaned from authorities in Camden to identify medical hotspots. Step two was to set up comprehensive health care for frequent flyers inside the hotspot.

"I can ride around the city and point to buildings and tell you how many people live in the building, how often they go the ER and hospital and why they go," says Brenner. "We went into one of those buildings and we opened a two-exam-room office right there. So patients can come down the elevator and be seen right in the building. About 100 patients in the building are coming down and the use of the clinic is really beginning to accelerate."

Step three in Brenner's plan was to set up a computer system that identifies patients who go to the ER to try to prevent return visits. "We pick patients up from the ER. We go to their house within twenty-four hours of an ER or hospital visit. We go with them to their primary-care appointment and with them to any key specialty appointments. We do a lot of training and education. It's a full-care coordination and management model."

How do they pay for this? For now, Brenner's group, Cooper University's Institute for Urban Health, has received a grant of $2.7 million to support the work of the Camden Coalition of Healthcare Professionals. If Brenner is right, the $2.7 million paid up front will translate into tens of millions of dollars of savings in the next five years. If successful, Brenner will have the ammunition he needs to approach state and federal governments to do this on a much larger scale. He calls it bending the health-care cost curve.

Preliminary evidence suggests the idea works. Remember Dennis Manners, the Louisville man who visited the ER at University Hospital 337 times in less than two years? The hospital enrolled Manners in its innovative Population Health Management Complex Case Program, which is patterned on what Brenner is doing in Camden. The results? The *Courier-Journal* reports that in the first eight months after Manners entered the program, he went to the ER just three times—far, far fewer than before. The cost of curtailing Manners's frequent visits: a paltry $6,000.

Half a continent away, Saskatoon's Dr. Ryan Meili is using the same idea but taking a somewhat different approach. In 2005, Meili helped found Student Wellness Initiative Toward Community Health (SWITCH), a storefront clinic run by health-care students that meets the needs of would-be frequent flyers. It's a block away from the ER at St. Paul's Hospital, the place Meili and the students want their patients to avoid.

Aside from paid administrative support people, volunteer health-care students staff the clinic—among them budding physicians, physiotherapists, nurses, dietitians and social workers. The idea behind the clinic is quite different from ER and hospital medicine. In the ER, we diagnose and treat clinical problems and ignore the social factors that contribute to the problem. At SWITCH, they treat medical problems but then pivot to social factors—issues such as housing, nutrition, immunizations and employment.

The difference begins right in the waiting room. In the ER, we don't like frequent flyers using the waiting room as a hangout. Unless it's the coldest night of the year, we actively encourage them to leave the moment their medical issues have been addressed. Not so at SWITCH, where the waiting area is a warm, inviting place for frequent flyers to hang out all day long. It even provides meals.

"We want people to come and stay and stay connected," says Meili. "At SWITCH, it's not just come and stay, but bring your kids. We have child care here, so that people participating in the programming or seeing the clinical team can have their kids taken care of."

Meili told me about a typical patient I'll call Rachel. "She was really struggling with anxiety problems," says Meili. "Lots of people would just stay in the waiting room and visit but she wanted to see the clinical team. So a medical student and a social work student went in and saw her first. They sat with this young woman, who shared her story and got a chance to tell them what she'd been struggling with. At the end of that visit, she started to cry and said she'd never had somebody listen to her in that depth. "I think this is a model that could really be expanded beyond a training centre like this to models of primary care."

What Meili and Brenner are trying to accomplish is something Brenner calls disruptive change. "What we really need in health care right now are delivery-system game changers that dramatically lower costs. And disruptive innovation, by its very nature, disrupts people's careers, disrupts their lives and fundamentally changes how you think about a problem."

In 2012, the U.S. Centers for Medicare and Medicaid Services announced it would start withholding up to 1 percent of Medicare payments from hospitals with too many frequent flyers. The maximum penalty is slated to rise to 3 percent by the year 2014. In the first year alone, the federal government is expected to dock more than 2,000 hospitals across the nation an estimated $280 million in Medicare payments. Medicare assembled the list of hospitals by looking at the thirty-day hospital readmission rate for patients with pneumonia, heart attack and congestive heart failure.

If frequent flyers like these could land at one of Jeffrey Brenner's clinics, they'd be better off. But in the absence of a program like Brenner's, it's far more likely that hospitals penalized for taking care of frequent flyers will give them an even chillier reception than they already receive.

Suffice it to say that in the absence of disruptive change, frequent flyers won't be going away any time soon. There's a weird thing about that. ER doctors like me are acculturated to dislike frequent flyers. The frustration we feel at their repeat visits can lead to potentially dangerous situations.

ER nurse Megen Duffy says, "Nobody really even makes an effort to be civil to these people. We're not rude to them, but it concerns me because we no longer take anything they say seriously, and at some point they're likely to be sick. Everybody actually has an emergency at some point in their lives and we might miss it because we see them so often with made-up complaints."

I'll never forget the last time I saw Donald. At the time, nothing seemed particularly special about that visit. As always, he came in with an anxious look in his eyes. He complained of pain in his chest and upper abdomen. It was quiet enough in the ER for me to sit with him while we waited for his heart tests to come back. I asked Donald about his wife. He spoke at length about her devotion to him and how he missed her.

Either he was grateful for some extra attention or perhaps it was something else. On this one occasion, when I told him that his heart tests were normal and bade him goodbye, he said something to me he'd never said before. "God bless you," said Donald, calmer than he had been when he arrived. Then he turned and walked out of the ER through the sliding doors.

A week later, I heard that Donald was found dead in his bed at home. I don't know if he perished from a heart attack that I missed, or if he died of a heart broken by the loneliness of widowhood. Instantly, his last words to me echoed in my mind. I had always felt disconnected from frequent flyers, a state of mind I suspect most of us who work in the ER have. Donald's words changed that forever. Every time I think of the patients I secretly mocked and ridiculed, I feel ashamed.

To me, they are no longer frequent flyers—just people in the wrong place. And one day, if people like Jeff Brenner have their way, there will be a lot fewer of them.

CHAPTER ELEVEN

Blocking and Turfing

'*ve introduced you to medical slang doctors use to describe patients a good many of us find undesirable—including GOMERs, Yellow Submarines and those with a bad case of status dramaticus. Those are examples of slang doctors and nurses share freely not just with trusted associates but with those who work on other teams—generalist and specialist alike. As a profession, doctors recognize that when it comes to difficult patients, they are the enemy and we—no matter what we specialize in—are on the same team.

Now I'm going to let you in on a different kind of medical argot—a form of slang that refers not to unwanted patients but to the things doctors do to avoid looking after them. This slang also describes the games doctors play to persuade colleagues to take undesirable patients off their hands. The trick is to manipulate the other doctors without acting or sounding manipulative. It's tricky.

Before I introduce the slang, check out this made-up but otherwise very typical conversation I have from time to time in the ER (usually around 1 a.m.) with a resident in internal medicine, in which I try to refer to his service an 87-year-old woman I'll call Mrs. Jones.

"Mrs. Jones has a history of hypertension, hypercholesterolemia and type 2 diabetes with associated chronic kidney disease," I tell the resident. (She has high blood pressure and high cholesterol, in addition to diabetes and kidney disease.) "She developed flu-like symptoms two days ago, including a cough now productive of sputum. Her daughter brought her to the ER because she was complaining of shortness of breath. Mrs. Jones felt feverish at home but didn't take her temperature. On physical examination, she is afebrile [without fever] with an oxygen saturation of 89 percent on room air, rising to 92 percent on three litres per minute of oxygen by nasal prongs. Her vitals are stable. On chest exam, she's got crackles on the right side. The rest of her examination is unremarkable. The chest X-ray looks like there's an early pneumonia on the right side. I've started her on intravenous moxifloxacin for the pneumonia."

"It might be an early pneumonia," the resident repeats my words with a note of skepticism. "What did the radiologist say?"

"The film hasn't been read yet," I reply.

"Do you mind asking the radiology resident to look at it?" the resident asks.

"I'm happy to ask the radiology resident to comment on the X-rays. But I'd still like you to see the patient."

"Why do you think she needs to be admitted?"

"As I said, I think she has pneumonia. She needs admission because her oxygen saturation was low on room air and improved on supplemental oxygen. That's why she's short of breath."

"What's the d-dimer?" the resident asks. A d-dimer is a blood test that can help rule out a pulmonary embolus (we nickname it PE), a blood clot on the lungs.

"I didn't order a d-dimer because I don't think she has a PE," I reply. "Mrs. Jones's symptoms are clearly those of a pneumonia-like illness, not a blood clot."

"What's her creatinine?" he asks. A serum creatinine is an important blood test that helps measure a patient's kidney function. The higher the serum creatinine level, the worse the kidney function.

"Her creatinine is 158," I tell the resident. In Canada, creatinine levels are expressed in SI units (measurements based on a modern form of the metric system) as micromoles per litre. In the United States, Mrs. Jones's creatinine would translate into a level of 1.79 milligrams per decilitre. Whichever units you prefer, Mrs. Jones had a creatinine level consistent with moderate kidney disease.

"Have you consulted nephrology?" the resident asks, referring to the specialty that deals with diseases of the kidney

"I don't think that's necessary at this time," I reply. "As I said, Mrs. Jones has chronic kidney disease caused by type 2 diabetes. She doesn't need dialysis. If you want to get a nephrology consult, be my guest."

"Did you do a lactate?" the resident asks me. A serum lactate is a blood test whose results are elevated in patients with sepsis, a potentially life-threatening complication of pneumonia and other infections.

"I didn't do a lactate because I don't think Mrs. Jones has sepsis," I reply, getting a bit impatient. "She has no fever and her vital signs are normal. If you want me to order a lactate, I'll be happy to do so, but I'd still like you to see the patient."

"If she has no fever, why can't she go home?" the resident asks.

"As I said, her oxygen saturation is low and she needs supplemental oxygen, which she can't get at home," I reply. By now I'm resisting the urge to ask the resident how may hours of sleep he had last night.

"What was her troponin?" he asks. A troponin is a highly sensitive blood test that measures certain proteins in the blood; it's ordered routinely to rule out a heart attack. Unfortunately, the troponin level is also elevated in patients with chronic kidney disease, like Mrs. Jones.

"Her troponin is 72 nanograms per litre," I reply, knowing what's coming next.

"That's a high troponin," notes the resident. "She could be having an ACS." (ACS stands for acute coronary syndrome, or heart attack.)

"But she has chronic kidney disease," I say. "That's probably the reason she has a high troponin. Her electrocardiogram showed no signs of an ACS."

"Still, that sounds more like a cardiology referral to me," says the resident, who turns and walks away.

I sigh. I've just spent ten minutes trying to sell a referral to an internal medicine resident young enough to be my son. I page the cardiology resident and repeat the story to her. By now, it is 3 a.m.

"Sounds like pneumonia to me," says the cardiology resident. "I'm happy to see the patient, but with her chronic kidney disease, I think internal medicine should admit her."

After I speak with the cardiology resident, I chat with the resident in internal medicine a second time.

"Why don't you get a repeat troponin?" he asks. "If it's not any higher than the first one, then I'll be happy to see her."

The second troponin level comes back from the lab at 6 a.m. I go back to see the internal medicine resident in a side room, where I find him seated with the other residents and students on his team.

"The second troponin is 70 nanograms per litre," I tell him. The second troponin level is just a hair less than the first test result, confirming that the elevated troponin level is caused by Mrs. Jones's kidney disease and not a heart attack. This is the proof the resident said he needed to accept Mrs. Jones onto his service. But that isn't the way things turn out.

"Oh, too bad," the resident says. "We're just about to go on rounds with our attending physician. I'm afraid the consult will have to wait until the new team comes on at eight o'clock."

As they say in tennis: Game, Set and Match. As I leave the room, I overhear one of the residents congratulate the team on blocking an admission. From the congratulatory tone, there is no thought whatsoever given to the fact that it will be another four hours until Mrs. Jones gets admitted to a bed, and her daughter—who has stayed up all night waiting to speak with the doctor who would be treating her mother—will finally be able to get some sleep.

//////

What that story illustrates is known in hospital lingo as blocking an admission—the resident in internal medicine stopped Mrs. Jones from being admitted to his service, hoping to leave the problem to another department.

Blocking is one term for patient avoidance; *turfing* is another. To turf a patient is to take a patient already admitted to one service and punt them to another. My favourite internal medicine resident, Dr. Nathan Stall, remembers hearing those words in an emergency room.

"I was with this emergency doctor and we were examining someone who had lower-limb weakness. He said he was just going to 'punt this patient to neurology.' The emergency physician got up, made a kicking motion as if he were kicking a football, in front of the patient and the family, and then walked out."

To get patients ready for turfing to another service, the admitting team needs to clean up any obvious lingering medical problems. If patients are dehydrated, they're given a bag of IV fluid to rehydrate them. If they're anemic, they're given a transfusion to bump up their hemoglobin. In slang terms, that's known as *buffing* the patient.

Sometimes, the team that receives the turfed patient punts the patient back to the original team. That's known in hospital parlance as a bounceback. A fourth term you hear in hospitals is *dumping* a patient from one service to another. Think of a dump as a flagrant or egregious turf. The patient is considered undesirable by the admitting team, which manages to turf the patient to another team, which finds the patient just as undesirable.

These terms aren't found in medical textbooks. But every doctor and nurse who works in a hospital has heard them and has a sense of what they mean—thanks to the slangmeister himself, Dr. Stephen Bergman.

In *The House of God*, the senior resident known as The Fat Man explains what a turf is to an intern named Potts. "To TURF is to get rid of, to get off your service and onto another, or out of the House altogether. Key concept. It's the main form of treatment in medicine."

And where did Bergman learn the word? I was startled to find out that he and his fellow interns invented it at Boston's Beth Israel Hospital in the early 1970s.

"I codified it," says Bergman. "I wrote about *buff* and *turf* and then, as I always do, I took it further. I'm sure I thought of the *bounce*—you know, when you turf a patient somewhere else and you haven't buffed him enough so he bounces back to you."

And the words flowed like a river from the slangmeister's pen to the lips of residents from generation to generation. Unlike many other bits of slang, *turfing, dumping* and *blocking* are known to all and done by everyone.

Dr. Nooreen Popat says she first heard these slang words when she was a resident in internal medicine at McMaster University in Hamilton, Ontario. "If you ask anyone who's a doctor they'll tell you they love their job," says Popat, who's now completing her training in respirology. "But sometimes in the middle of the night, when everything's really busy in the hospital, people are trying to do less work. So they may turf to one another or dump on one another and that was how I first came into contact with this. I was sort of surprised at what was going on and the connotation of the language that was being used."

I'm not surprised one bit. Unlike unacceptable slang such as *harpooning the whale*, words like *blocking, turfing* and *dumping* are known and used widely by administrators of hospitals and managed health-care plans, directors of residency programs and even by researchers as genuine phenomena to be studied and understood. In other words, they've become an institution.

Do a search on Medline, the database of the National Library of Congress, and you're certain to find them. In an article published in 2007 in the journal *Perspectives in Biological Medicine,* Dr. Catherine Caldicott, an internist and bioethicist, wrote that turfing is a "widespread phenomenon in medical training programs."

One of the experts trying to understand what words like these mean and what and how they reflect on the culture of modern medicine is Dr. Vineet Arora. Associate program director for the Internal Medicine Residency at the University of Chicago, she is one of the bright lights in the emerging field of medical professionalism. Arora and her colleagues set out to determine just how commonly the tug-of-war between the ER and other services takes place. "We asked students and residents if they occur in the workplace and they all said they do," says Arora. "And they all recognized the terms *blocking* and *turfing.*"

Because *The House God*—the original manual of turfology, if we can call it that—was a novel about junior doctors, one might assume that they are the only practitioners of turfing. Surely attending physicians don't do that sort of thing.

Oh, but they do. Arora co-wrote a study published in 2012 in the *Journal of Hospital Medicine* that surveyed unprofessional behaviour among hospitalists, doctors who practise in hospitals. Nearly 8 percent said they had participated in blocking an admission to hospital and more than 9 percent said they had participated in turfing a patient to another service. A much higher percentage of hospitalists surveyed said they'd witnessed blocking and turfing by colleagues.

Arora says you need inside knowledge to execute a turf. "People that had administrative jobs like running the clinical service (supervising residents on the wards) were more likely to engage in those behaviours," says Arora. "That really highlights the fact that you're unlikely to be able to block and turf if you don't know how the system works. I think that it's something you see more with senior residents and attending physicians."

Even more disturbing is the fact that 21 percent of respondents in Arora's study said they had celebrated a blocked admission and nearly 12 percent had celebrated a successful turf.

When it comes to turfing and blocking, there are winners and there are losers. That's what is going on in the minds of many residents and a surprising number of attending physicians too. It's about aggressors foisting their unwanted patients on someone else.

Blocking a referral during a night on call is one payoff. Bragging about it to your colleagues the next morning is another. Dr. Nathan Stall says boasting happens a lot. "I've shown up in the morning and that's being thrown around," he says. "'You had one consult and sent back four last night. *Wow*, that's impressive,' is what colleagues will say. 'Nice work. Now the team only has to pick up one new patient. Less work for everybody else [on the team].'"

⁄⁄⁄⁄⁄⁄⁄

About a decade ago, organized medicine invented the phrase *patient-centred care*. In a 2001 report titled *Crossing the Quality Chasm: A New Health System for the 21st Century*, the Institute of Medicine (IOM) defined patient-centred care as "health care that establishes a partnership among practitioners, patients, and their families (when appropriate) to ensure that decisions respect patients' wants, needs, and preferences and that patients have the education and support they need to make decisions and participate in their own care."

The IOM is one of the most respected medical institutions in the world. Established in 1970, the IOM is the health arm of the National Academy of Sciences, which was founded in 1863, when Abraham Lincoln was president of the United States. To me, the very fact that the IOM felt the need to articulate something as obvious as patient-centred care serves notice that the culture of modern medicine has other priorities in mind.

Think of it. You come to the hospital with chest pain, trouble breathing, or some blood in your bowel movements. Or maybe you bring your mother or your father with a cracked pelvis or a broken hip caused by a fall. The first doctor you see is an ER physician like me. I take a history, do a physical examination and order some tests. If I think you need admission to hospital, I call the appropriate attending physician.

From your vantage point in an ER cubicle, the attending or the resident comes to see you, agrees to accept you, and off you go to a bed upstairs on the wards. But from what I've told you about turfing, dumping, buffing and bounce-backs, the picture I just painted is anything but patient centred.

While you or a loved one wait to be admitted to hospital, just a few metres away from your cubicle, yet well outside of earshot, physicians may be verbally duking it out over your immediate future. The aim is not so much to care for you as to find a clever way to jettison that responsibility by finding someone else to do it.

Let's take a closer look at what might make you or your loved one undesirable. The likeliest candidate for turfing is any patient who isn't young, or interesting in a clinical or diagnostic sense. Often it's a patient who can no longer live independently. Being unable to control your bodily fluids is another strike against you.

The thing is, you or your loved one can't go home. You need to be admitted to hospital. To get an internist to admit you, the trick is to make you look as sexy as possible in a diagnostic sense. Often I play up a patient's clinical issues, such as low serum sodium or a slight increase in their liver tests, to get the internist to say yes. In medical slang, we call that *making the sale.*

"You get a referral in which fictitious medical problems are made up to justify seeing the patient," says Nooreen Popat. "You discover there are no real medical problems but there are some social issues, and they just can't go home. So that could be kind of like a dump."

Turfs or dumps—whatever you call them—involve two parties: the doctor or team transferring the patient and the one receiving the patient. Of course, the patient makes three, but in the give-and-take of hospital admissions, patients are often little more than passive participants—no matter how much their lives are on the line.

This phenomenon exposes a secret about the culture of modern medicine that few outsiders appreciate. When patients are being shopped around, different kinds of specialists view each other with deep suspicion—especially surgeons and internists. Just ask Dr. Andrew Burke, a resident in internal medicine.

"My 'Spidey sense' starts to tingle when another specialty service—for example, general surgery—says a patient is more appropriate for me but will not mention anything related to the gastrointestinal or the abdominal or any of the areas that they normally specialize in. So you can just kind of tell that's being played down. It's all about emphasis. That's when you start to smell a hint of a turf," says Burke.

There is a rough division of labour between internists and general surgeons. The surgeons admit patients with abdominal pain caused by conditions that often but not always require an operation. Appendicitis, inflamed gall bladder and bowel cancers immediately come to mind. Internists admit patients with non-surgical conditions. They don't want each other's patients because they don't want to tie up a hospital bed that could be used to admit someone more appropriate.

But that's not all. Though they seldom admit it, internists and surgeons alike feel lost at sea caring for each other's patients—and are terrified such patients will die on their watch. An internal medicine resident remembers a patient with a complicated history of internal medicine problems who would ordinarily have been referred to an internist on call. But because the patient had abdominal pain, a referral was made to a surgeon.

"Then I got a call from the surgery team a few hours later saying they wanted me to see the patient," the resident recalls. "They said it seemed like the patient had an infection [as opposed to a surgical condition] and could I look after him?"

The surgeons didn't talk about the patient's abdominal pain or get into the reasons the surgeons were asked to see the patient in the first place.

"Foolishly, I said I would go see the patient, no problem," she says. "As it turned out, two or three hours later, the patient actually needed to go to the OR urgently."

Fortunately, one of the junior residents on her team was experienced in surgery and recognized that the patient urgently needed an operation. She says they were able to persuade the surgeons to take the patient back in time to save his life.

It was only after the fact that the resident learned exactly why the surgeons had turfed the patient to her team.

"What I found out is that the surgeons had another urgent OR case," she says. "The surgery team didn't want to take care of a patient that they didn't know [for certain] was surgical, so they turfed it to us. That way, they could go deal with something that they knew was surgical. But that was a turf that could have gone wrong."

The most dangerous examples are turfs in which the turfing physicians omit critical details or even lie about the patient's condition to make the sale. This is often true when a doctor working at a small community hospital requests that a patient be transferred to a major urban referral centre.

A different resident in internal medicine remembers the time she received a referral from a physician who said his patient was having a heart attack. When the patient arrived by ambulance, it was clear to the resident that the patient was not having a heart attack but was suffering from a life-threatening infection called sepsis. In the resident's view, the referring physician underplayed the gravity of the patient's condition to guarantee that the patient would be accepted for transfer. "That was an example of buffing or shining up a patient," she says.

Sometimes the referring physician does the exact opposite and executes a turf by overplaying the gravity of the patient's condition to make it seem more urgent than it really is. "They'll say the patient has chest pain at rest," says the resident. Chest pain that occurs while a patient is at rest might indicate an impending heart attack.

"That's a red flag that tells us we need to run and see the patient," she adds. "When you get there, you realize it was an exaggeration on the part of the person handing the patient over because they wanted you to take the patient."

Sometimes, the tensions between physicians on competing admitting teams can run so high that fights actually break out.

"I've seen a cardiac surgeon and an ICU doctor screaming at the top of their lungs as to who was going to take a patient," says a recent graduate who was in his final year of med school when he witnessed the argument. "Then one of them turned to the other—and there's family members in there and a young person dying—saying, 'Do you want to take this outside?' I couldn't believe it. It was so childish."

Stories like these keep Dr. Vineet Arora awake at night.

"When you start blocking or turfing, you're engaging in a long battle for a marginal patient that it's easier for you to keep," she says. "When you're engaging in that long battle, time is passing. What often happens is that the patient gets worse because nobody is paying attention to them because they're too fixated on where the patient should go in all that blocking and turfing."

A big part of Arora's interest in turfing, blocking and dumping is the risk posed to the safety of patients. Arora, who analyzes the root causes of medical mistakes, says she makes a point of asking doctors involved in medical mistakes if the time spent blocking a referral caused the patient to suffer.

"The answer is almost always yes."

⁄⁄⁄⁄⁄⁄⁄

Why has a form of behaviour introduced in Bergman's novel evolved into such a problem? The answer is a mélange of issues to do with the health-care system as well as personality factors common in people who become physicians.

In the U.S., patients who are a financial drain on a hospital are at risk of being turfed or dumped elsewhere. It doesn't seem to matter whether the hospital is private, Medicare and Medicaid, or part of a managed health-care system.

For instance, it's been said that these shenanigans happen mainly in teaching hospitals, where doctors are on salary as opposed to getting a fee per admission, so they aren't that motivated to accept new patients. By contrast, in private practices doctors get a fee for each patient, which provides an incentive to see the patients that docs in teaching hospitals turf. But that's not the way it goes.

In her paper published in *Virtual Medicine*, Dr. Catherine Caldicott, the turfing expert from Denver, Colorado, wrote: "It is not unusual for private practices to decline patients with Medicare, Medicaid, or no medical insurance and refer them to the nearest academic center." That sounds a lot like dumping patients to me.

The practice has been so widespread in the U.S. that in 1986, a federal law called the Emergency Medical Treatment and Labor Act was passed to prevent hospitals from turning away patients with emergency medical conditions.

Even so, a 2012 article published in the journal *Health Affairs* shows that twenty-five years after the law was passed, patient blocking and dumping continue largely unimpeded. The article focused on Denver Health, a highly integrated health-care system, which has experienced a steady growth in the care of uninsured patients, much of it provided at Denver Health Medical Center. Among the charges, the article documented the fact that other hospitals were discharging unstable patients and specialists were refusing to treat uninsured patients. In April 2013, Nevada Governor Brian Sandoval was forced to defend his state after a report that psychiatric hospitals in Las Vegas sent hundreds of discharged patients by bus to California and other states.

The system of managed health care has also increased the temptation to turf, according to Peter Kongstvedt, an authority on the health-care industry, health insurance and managed care. In his book *The Managed Health Care Handbook*, Kongstvedt describes a doctor who removed sick patients from his practice. Since sick patients require more tests and treatments, removing them makes the doctor appear not to overuse health services.

Dr. Caldicott says some of what appears to be turfing behaviour may not be that at all. She says the U.S. health-care system is so fragmented and complex that most doctors who work in it feel pressure to move patients through the system as quickly and as efficiently as possible. "I think most physicians feel constrained to do only a small thing every time they see a patient and only think narrowly and only answer the one specific question," Caldicott said in an interview, "because there are so many pressures to see a large number of patients in a short amount of time and to make the bean counters happy."

But this is not just a product of a dysfunctional U.S. health-care system. Turfing, dumping and blocking of patient admissions are well known to physicians in Canada. I had no trouble finding residents north of the forty-ninth parallel to dish stories on the phenomenon.

Financial issues may explain the practice of turfing and dumping between hospitals. What they don't answer is why such horse-trading goes on between doctors who work at the *same* hospital. That has more to do with individual factors such as resident fatigue.

Onerous work hours were once thought to be the reason residents block admissions and turf patients. But the trouble with that argument is that the past few years have seen resident duty hours cut fairly dramatically. If long duty hours were the main factor that encouraged turfing and dumping, then the problem should be in the rear-view mirror.

Unfortunately, it isn't. For one thing, I've spoken with many residents who choose not to leave when their shifts end. Residents in general surgery tell me they stay because they don't want to risk a bad evaluation from their attending surgeon. The ones who do leave when their duty hours are complete may be even more likely to block referrals near the end of their tour of duty because they don't want to have to work overtime taking care of the patient.

In a 2012 paper published in the journal *Virtual Mentor*, Catherine Caldicott expressed skepticism that reducing resident hours had any effect. "Despite the absence of hard data, anecdotal reports substantiate that turfing persists," she wrote.

Caldicott looked at turfing and dumping as issues of power between residents. In a revealing study published in 1999 in the *Journal of General Internal Medicine*, she and co-author Dr. David Stern analyzed audiotapes of residents' discussions on turfing and concluded that the language of turfing is born of emotions among residents in internal medicine. They wrote: "Residents can feel angry and frustrated about receiving patients seemingly rejected by other doctors, while feeling powerless to prevent the transfer of patients for whom they can offer neither effective treatment nor continuous relationship."

Dr. Vineet Arora is a mentor to residents. Not too many years removed from her own residency in internal medicine, Arora can still see things from their point of view. "As a resident, you have so little control over most of your life," she says. "If you're able to have control over the number of patients that you admit, that's at least something that you can say you did for yourself. It definitely happens and it's more likely to happen when people are burned out and lacking the systems to promote wellness and at the brink of being overworked."

One of the things I've noticed over the years is that turfing and blocking tend to ebb and flow with the arrival and departure of new residents. Why is that?

"All it takes is one bad egg for this to start occurring," Arora says. "Every residency has somebody that's known for blocking. People develop reputations. So if you know you're going to call a resident who has a reputation for blocking, you're going to make the patient sound as sick as possible to get accepted on the resident's service."

In *The House of God*, a resident with a good reputation for blocking admissions was known as a wall. And it's not just residents who develop such reputations. "I work with hospitalists and we see this behaviour in hospitalists too," says Arora.

Catherine Caldicott says the bad egg Arora was talking about might even be an attending physician. "Where do you think the residents learn it from?" she asks rhetorically. "I remember hearing and seeing residents doing high fives over turfing a patient and having the attending bring the team a case of beer to celebrate not taking a patient on their service."

In turn, those residents grow up into attending physicians and teach that sort of behaviour to their residents. And so it goes.

///////

In some instances, it's actually in a patient's best interest to get transferred from one hospital or hospital ward to another. There are days when the internist or the team of residents on call admits as many as 30 patients. That's a lot of new and acutely ill patients to workup and possibly misdiagnose and mistreat.

"You're basically guarding against more work for your team because you know you're already at the tipping point where you may actually be very unsafe," says Arora.

And sometimes, a patient is admitted to hospital by a surgeon who, after looking for a surgical problem, discovers there isn't one.

"Let's say there's a patient I'm taking care of who is no longer interesting to me," says Dr. Christopher Kinsella, a resident in general surgery in St. Louis. "They don't need surgery but they're sick. The patient needs to be in a hospital, and needs to be taken care of by someone. The last thing you want is to have a patient being taken care of by doctors who are no longer interested in that patient."

True enough, but sometimes the turfing happens only once the surgeon has operated on the patient, who has not gotten any better.

Now the patient's diabetes and high blood pressure are getting worse. And the patient is getting sicker and sicker. Slowly, it dawns on the attending physician that the patient may not make it out of the hospital alive.

In an era of managed health care and increased accountability for results, a death on your service looks bad and may result in financial penalties for the attending physician or surgeon as well as the hospital.

"And so they transfer the patient to a medical service so that the patient dies on medicine rather than on surgery so the [surgeon's] numbers look better," says Caldicott, quoting a belief often stated by attending physicians on the receiving end of such transfers. "I can't prove any of this at all, but you and I have both seen and heard people behave in ways that would make it sound like these things I'm saying are plausible."

/////////

In 2010, U.S. President Barack Obama signed into law the Affordable Care Act (ACA), complex health legislation that came to be known as Obamacare. Obamacare is the first substantive update on legislation related to the provision of health care in the U.S. since the introduction of Medicare in 1965. The legislation seeks to provide health insurance for 35 million of the 50 million Americans without it, making a step toward the type of universal coverage enjoyed by Canadians.

The ACA proposed to do that by expanding Medicaid. So far, twenty-six states are going ahead with the expansion, fifteen have opted out and the rest remain undecided.

Though it's too soon to gauge its full impact, the hope is that Obamacare will reduce the financial pressure to turf patients by increasing the number of insured Americans. There's some evidence that increasing the number of patients on Medicaid is improving accountability. The U.S. Centers for Medicare and Medicaid Services has the power to investigate and penalize hospitals that practice patient dumping.

These measures may help reduce turfing and dumping at the system level. But so much of the practice takes place between individual physicians. Fixing that requires a different approach.

Catherine Caldicott has called for educational workshops to teach doctors that turfing is unprofessional. If one medical student's experience is any indication, we have a lot of educating to do. During a rotation in surgery, the student remembers caring for a man in his fifties who was developmentally delayed and was living in assisted housing. The patient had been diagnosed with rectal cancer and had an ostomy pouch—an external bag—for his bowel movements. He arrived in the ER with abdominal pain and soon developed life-threatening problems that required emergency stabilization.

The man was critically ill, the student says, and the ER physician summoned a phalanx of residents in surgery, internal medicine, gastroenterology and the ICU to stabilize him. Then one of the residents took the family aside and asked them what they wanted for the patient.

"They decided that this gentleman with developmental delay had a hard life and that the rectal cancer hadn't been easy," says the student. "They didn't want anything done to him."

And with that, every resident who had been trying to save the man's life just walked away.

"No one wanted to take this patient on," the student adds. "I felt terrible."

Vineet Arora has no doubt what patients and their families would think about what was done to the student's patient. "They would think it's horrible," Arora says. "I would be embarrassed to tell a patient [about turfing and blocking]. I think that patients have a right to high-quality care. They are hoping that they just get a plan and get good care and get home safely. To not feel wanted is, of course, going to be tragic."

Given his role in introducing residents and medical students to terms like *blocking, turfing* and *buffing,* I wanted to know what author Stephen Bergman thinks of the fact that these concepts have become institutions in the culture of modern hospital medicine.

"The reality was that we would never turf a patient who we thought really needed our care," says Bergman, who is more than a little astonished that turfing has become such an institutional practice. He points out that what he wrote was a novel. "You can't let the jokes be the reality. You can't let the slang be the reality."

But turfing and dumping are the reality of modern medicine. Surprised though he may be, Stephen Bergman captured and reflected something in the attitude of residents and attending physicians back then. It's probably even worse today.

CHAPTER TWELVE

Cowboys and Fleas

B y now, you've grasped the notion that physicians and other health-care professionals use slang to tell each other just how much they dislike or—more charitably—feel frustrated treating certain kinds of patients. What you may not know is that their antipathy for colleagues also runs *very* deep. The myth of physicians and surgeons of various kinds riding off to war together to battle disease and injury—like the Knights of the Round Table—is just that: a myth.

Listen carefully inside the Bunker or at a nursing station late at night and you'll hear surgeons rip internists, internists moan about surgeons, residents complain about attending physicians and seemingly everyone diss family doctors and ER physicians like me.

"I think that doctor-to-doctor slang is probably a lot more brutal than doctor-to-patient slang because there's no confidentiality here," says Dr. Grumpy, the neurologist blogger. "The other doctor isn't sick and seeking help. It's just another person you have to deal with."

Dr. Grumpy says it's not uncommon to hear doctors refer to each other as "morons" and words that are much worse.

"Usually it's just plain insulting—like dipshit or dumb fuck or bozo," he says. "I think bozo is probably the most commonly used one. You try not to use that with patients. I've never used it directly with another doctor. Usually it's more in passing, where I'm looking over someone else's notes and I'm thinking, 'God, this guy is a bozo. What he's doing makes no sense.' I think it's pretty common."

Dr. Grumpy remembers using the term to describe a fellow neurologist who specialized in managing patients with headaches such as migraines. Dr. Grumpy says the doctor, who trained at a celebrated medical clinic in the U.S., opened an office near his and sent out a letter announcing the opening of the practice and asking for referrals. Dr. Grumpy decided to send one of his most hard-to-treat headache patients to see if the new doctor had any suggestions for how to control the patient's symptoms.

"He sent me back this incredibly crappy letter," Dr. Grumpy recalls. "He didn't give me any information on what medications I should use aside from telling me not to use the ones I had already tried. He suggested I do tests that had already been done. It was a remarkably worthless and unpleasant experience and the patient was horribly disappointed. She said she felt he was rude—obviously a bozo."

The way Dr. Grumpy talks about other doctors is pretty typical. It's embedded in the culture of medicine that one kind of doctor disses another.

"There's the joke about orthopedic wards being the place where internal medicine patients go to die," says Dr. Donovan Gray, an ER physician and author of *Dude, Where's My Stethoscope?*

Gray cites the oft-told story: A patient is admitted to an orthopedics ward for an operation to fix a broken foot bone. The patient also happens to have diabetes, but the orthopedic surgeon fails to diagnose or even recognize the symptoms of a diabetic emergency. "The orthopedic surgeon comes around to look at the foot and says that [it looks] good—and off he goes. Meanwhile, the patient's in a coma."

It's startling for outsiders to hear doctors talking about each other that way. I found it so when I first heard that sort of dissing during residency. That's when we learn the secret language of collegial insults. Now I'm used to it.

Five metres from your gurney or hospital bed, doctors discuss each other like that all the time. It's just that you never hear it. That's because complaining publicly about a colleague's clinical skill, judgment, competence and attentiveness is considered unethical— perhaps even a breach of professional conduct. Hospitals and physicians may be inching slowly toward coming clean and apologizing for medical mistakes. But the unofficial hospital code of behaviour says that if you've nothing good to say to a patient about a colleague, say nothing.

Your only clue that something's not right with your medical care may be found in the secret language we use to talk about each other.

⁄⁄⁄⁄⁄⁄⁄

The slang used by doctors to disparage each other may vary with the hospital. But certain terms are remarkably common.

Surgeons are cowboys. Internists are fleas. And ER physicians— like me—are often referred to derisively as "triage nurses." That's a rare example of slang that demeans not one but two colleagues—ER physicians and triage nurses—at the same time. And make no mistake: slang words like these are seldom compliments.

To begin to understand the meaning and the antipathy behind the slang, we need to go back to the origins of medical specialization. Although physicians had specialized since the time of the Romans, by the 1880s it was considered a necessity so that doctors could advance medical knowledge more quickly by observing many cases of only one or two diseases.

The unintended effect of specialization is that it created rivalries between specialists, born to a large extent out of insecurity. The more specialized doctors became, the less they knew about what each other did, and the more they had to depend upon fellow specialists who possessed skills they did not have and practices they knew increasingly little about, to help care for their patients. For decades, that insecurity bubbled under the surface. Then, in 1961, Peter Hukill and James Jackson co-wrote an article that was the first to capture argot or cant used by doctors to describe their colleagues. Most of it was pretty tame. Urologists were referred to as plumbers or as doctors whose specialty was the waterworks. Anesthesiologists were called gas passers, a slang term still used today.

"I find that an offensive term, and I would never use it in my practice," says Dr. Katherine Grichnik, professor of anesthesiology and critical-care medicine in the department of anesthesiology at Duke University Medical Center in Durham, North Carolina. As associate dean for continuing medical education in the Duke School of Medicine, Grichnik is a thought leader in the evolution of professionalism among physicians. "I would never use it with a patient and I would never allow a surgeon to say it to me because it's trivializing the profession."

To prove her point, Grichnik outlines the complex knowledge anesthesiologists acquire to deliver safe and effective anesthesia care. It involves mastering the latest anesthetic drugs and techniques for a growing number of increasingly sick patients with complex and burgeoning medical problems. Anesthesiologists also have to worry about "what the surgeon's going to do, and the complexities of the operation," adds Grichnik. "Passing gas doesn't convey any of that at all."

Her colleague Dr. Peter Kussin, a respirologist at Duke University Hospital, doesn't disagree with Grichnik; he just thinks slang isn't all that demeaning. Kussin, Duke's most notorious slangmeister, openly uses argot to refer to other specialists and he uses those terms with unconcealed delight.

Like pecker checkers—otherwise known as urologists.

Sometimes, Kussin springs slang like this on his residents just to see the looks on their faces. He recalls being on rounds in a medical intensive care unit and needing to know what urologists had said about a patient. He says he asked his team of residents, "Well, what do the pecker checkers think?

"Their eyes opened wide and I repeated: 'Have you talked to the pecker checkers?' One of the residents pointed behind me. I turned around and there was the senior urologist! And he says, 'Well, the pecker checkers are here, Peter.'

"We laughed because he was about my age, and it was okay," says Kussin.

Kussin has lots more where that one came from that he likes to teach his residents.

"The one they never know is *pitchforks*, which is one of my favourite slang terms for psychiatrists." Aside from the reference to the devil, the slang was completely lost on me until Kussin explained that the open end of a pitchfork looks a lot like the Greek letter *psi*, which in medical circles stands for psychiatry.

"I'll say, 'Get the pitchforks in' and my residents will say, 'What?'" says Kussin. "And I'll say, 'Get a psychiatry consult.' They love that because it's a pure symbolism, wordplay thing and it's very poetic."

///////

Poetic or crude, the slang doctors use in hospital to talk about each other serves an important yet largely unspoken purpose: it reinforces a kind of tribalism.

We enter medical school as equals. We take the same courses and pass the same exams. But then we enter the various residencies. And by the time we're finished with that part of our training, we belong to a tribe of "Us" separated from all other tribes, to be regarded forever as "Them."

For example, ER physicians like me see internists and surgeons not as colleagues but as people we have to persuade to accept the patients we refer to them. When they give us a hard time by asking too many questions, we get our backs up. We get defensive. Often, we feel humiliated. In the same way, we see radiologists as people who have the power to say yes or no to that CT scan of the abdomen we need to diagnose appendicitis or at the very least to cover our butts by proving to an anxious and possibly litigious patient that she has nothing serious going on inside her belly. In our worst moments, we see radiologists as doctors who don't practise real medicine because they sit in a dark room all day looking at pictures.

At the same time, internists, surgeons and radiologists don't see ER physicians and other specialists as their equals in medical knowledge and in the ability to make diagnoses that they find easy but people like me find difficult. Sometimes, different specialists see each other as competitors for patients and sometimes even as adversaries.

Cardiologists may feel superior to internists just as neurosurgeons think they're a cut above their less-trained "colleagues" who take out your appendix. They believe they're a much higher form of primate in the hospital zoo. Family doctors and ER physicians feel insecure and inferior next to their specialist colleagues. And residents often feel abused and persecuted by their attending physicians. The slang doctors use to describe each other only symbolizes the differences among us. Money, power and influence are the envy factors that reinforce those differences.

In his 2008 book *Us and Them: The Science of Identity*, author David Berreby says humans are hard-wired to form connections with one another based on trivial commonalities; Berreby calls that ability "kind sight." What's astonishing is that the seeds of the vast differences between groups of physicians can be found in those tiny commonalities. Kind sight is in our human nature because it was once necessary for our very survival. It's difficult to argue that sort of motivation should exist between surgeons and internists in the twenty-first-century hospital. But it does.

It comes out in the way doctors talk—especially the slang we use to describe each other. This sort of talk goes on everywhere doctors and other health professionals ply their trade, from the lowly clinic in rural Arkansas to the most sophisticated of tertiary-care facilities.

In addition to serving up some of the most well-respected health care in the U.S., one hospital I visited serves up something else: a healthy dose of medical slang—some of it used to describe colleagues in less than flattering terms.

The anesthesia residents' lounge there doesn't look like much; a three-by-five-metre room with a desk, a couple of desktop computers, a printer, two sofas and some chairs. Still, it's a refuge where residents in anesthesia can relax between cases in the OR—and grouse about their surgical colleagues on the other side of the surgical drape.

"Portraying the surgeons as butchers or carpenters or mechanics is probably not unfair," says a third-year resident in anesthesiology.

I'm seldom shocked to hear that sort of rush to judgment from residents like the two anesthesiologists I spoke to at this particular hospital. But I was more than a bit surprised to hear something similar from an experienced attending physician.

It's 8 a.m., and I'm attending rounds in one of the hospital's intensive care units. There are sixteen rooms—each containing a very sick patient decked out with a ventilator, a urinary catheter, one or two central venous lines, an arterial line and some plain old intravenous drips as well. A veteran attending specialist in critical-care medicine is leading a large and unwieldy pack of seventeen health professionals, including residents, nurses, speech therapists, a registered dietitian and a respiratory therapist. Rounds are a daily ritual in which the team discusses extraordinarily complex care plans that keep the patients alive.

"The patient's vitals are stable and so is his urine output," says a senior ICU resident who acts as second-in-command. "He still has a nasogastric tube in. He's got so much suction coming back I think we can kill the Lasix."

Translation: The patient is doing well except for the fact that he has a poorly functioning bowel that is causing his intestines and his bloodstream to fill up with fluids—so much so that he was given the powerful diuretic Lasix to keep his lungs from filling up with water. Now he's becoming dehydrated and the resident wants to discontinue the Lasix.

Up to that point, the resident has spoken about the technical patois of critical care. Suddenly, he adds an observation that pricks up my ears. "The vascular surgeon decided to put the patient on some chicken heparin," he says. Members of the group smile.

I'm quite sure no doctor anywhere—much less the highly respected ones who practise at this top-flight centre—administer any medicines to patients that are derived from poultry. It sure sounds like slang to me. I pull aside the attending physician for a translation.

Chicken heparin is a term used "when the surgeons are too chicken to fully anticoagulate the patient," says the ICU attending physician.

To anticoagulate means to give the patient a medication like heparin to make the blood less likely to clot. The meds are called blood thinners and they're used to prevent patients who have had surgery from forming blood clots in the legs that can travel to the lungs and cause a potentially fatal complication called pulmonary embolus.

The ICU attending physician was accusing the surgeon of ordering a dose of heparin too low to actually prevent clots. "They want the patient's blood not to clot but they're afraid to go all the way."

Spying the chicken surgeon in a corridor of the ICU, the attending doctor steps away from the team to confront him about the order for chicken heparin. After five minutes, she comes back with a wide grin on her face.

"I told him I'd like to see the data supporting the use of low-dose heparin," she triumphantly tells the assembled team. "He replied, 'There is no data.' Asking people for data is the polite way to ask what the heck they're doing," she adds with a smile.

As a sincere inquiry, asking for data is part of sharing the latest medical knowledge. But asking for data when you already know that there is none is code for "You don't know what you're talking about."

The message was not lost on the ICU team. The attending looked smart and prudent; the vascular surgeon looked foolish. That sort of petty rivalry is not unique to this particular hospital. And if that sort of talk happens there, believe me, it happens everywhere.

/////////

In their 1961 article, Hukill and James were among the first to hint at the emerging rivalry between internists and surgeons. The authors noted that a specialist in internal medicine was known back then as a pill pusher, in sharp contrast to a surgeon. Clearly, the term *pill pusher* was used by surgeons to dismiss the work done by their colleagues in internal medicine. And, just as clearly, non-surgeons got in a little dig at their surgical colleagues. The phrase *knife-happy* made it onto the list compiled in the 1961 article. Analogous to trigger-happy, *knife-happy* refers to a surgeon who is overeager to take a patient to the operating room.

"The rivalry between surgeons and non-surgeons goes back," says Dr. Grumpy. "I mean it's even mentioned in the Hippocratic Oath. It's old."

You can't talk about the rivalries between various kinds of physicians without talking about the money they make. According to a 2012 survey by Medscape/Web M.D., the top U.S. medical money earners on average were radiologists and orthopedic surgeons at $315,000 a year each; cardiologists earned $314,000 a year, with anesthesiologists and urologists rounding out the list of high rollers at $309,000 a year.

At the other end of the scale, psychiatrists earned $170,000, diabetes specialists $168,000 and internists $165,000, followed by family doctors at $158,000 and pediatricians at $156,000.

There is no doubt that the higher the pay, the greater the respect—often grudging—among colleagues. And let's not forget the envy that doctors feel toward other physicians who make a lot more money than we do. Income is the lightning rod for medical argot about competence and work habits of physicians.

You've heard of the road to success? Dr. Ryan Madanick, a gastroenterologist at the University of North Carolina School of Medicine in Chapel Hill, says the acronym ROAD has become a telling slang word in medicine. It stands for "radiology, ophthalmology and orthopedic surgery, anesthesiology and dermatology."

"Those five fields are the road to financial success," says Madanick. They are also targets of professional envy. "This is especially true among internists, family practitioners, pediatricians, psychiatrists [and] OBGYNs: that you go into a field like dermatology, and the same with radiology, because it's easy work and it's lots of money. I'm not going to say that other groups don't work, but they get less financial remuneration for their mental work or for the time that they put in. I would certainly love to make the money that they do for the amount of time that they put in per patient per procedure or what have you, but it's not the field I chose."

Peter Kussin says he refers to rheumatologists as ruminologists, because they ruminate, and dermatologists as dermaholidays. "I think a lot of it has to do with workload. The lighter the perceived workload of a specialty, the more ribbing they'll take and the more slang that will be directed at them."

I think Kussin is right. When I did rotations in rheumatology and dermatology, I was rarely on call and always got a good night's sleep. We called those slack rotations.

The rivalry between groups of physicians is a natural reflection of our competitive personalities. In med school, it's all about who gets the top marks. Then we graduate.

"All of sudden, you're in a job or a specialty or a practice," Kathy Grichnik says. "How do you continue to achieve? How can I make myself better? Unfortunately, the historical culture has based this on 'getting better marks' than another physician."

Getting marks ends with medical school; the drive to establish superiority over colleagues can last a lifetime. Income, a stock portfolio, a Ferrari in driveway or a yacht parked at the marina is the attending doctor's equivalent for top of the class.

But there may be more to the sniping than envy and competitiveness. Sometimes it reflects genuine concerns about another physicians' competence.

One doctor I know refers to that sort of criticism as a "back-channel M and M." *M and M* is slang for the morbidity and mortality conferences held regularly in hospitals to discuss cases in which concerns have been raised that a poor patient outcome (death or injury) was caused by suboptimal medical care. The conferences originated in the early twentieth century at the Massachusetts General Hospital in Boston. At M and Ms, the case is discussed anonymously and without blaming or punishing the people involved. The objective is to discover mistakes and correct them so as to prevent them from happening again.

"It's an ongoing M and M where we comment on their foibles and they comment on our foibles," says my colleague. "This is a way of us maintaining sort of back-channel quality control."

Unspoken or not, reputations matter in all walks of life—including medicine. Every clinical ward has a jungle telegraph that tells us what we think about the reliability, bedside manner and—last but not least—the clinical acumen and competence of our colleagues and everyone else we rely on when we're taking care of you.

A 1993 article in the journal *Social Science & Medicine* by Robert Coombs and colleagues referred to Gomer Doc and Fossil Doc as physicians who haven't kept up with recent medical developments. An HST refers to an uptight attending physician with "high sphincter tone"—a tight-ass. A private physician with a bad reputation for killing patients is known as Double O Private—a riff on the Ian Fleming character James Bond, code name 007, who famously has a licence to kill.

To appreciate that part of hospital culture, a good way to begin is to pick up on the slang.

////////

One of the most enduring bits of medical argot doctors use in less-than-flattering ways is calling each other "cowboy." The quintessential cowboy used to be a general surgeon. Today, surgeons of all kinds can earn the label.

"A cowboy is someone who rides by the seat of his pants," says

Dr. Grumpy. "It's someone who kind of does things quickly. You're trying hurriedly to do everything in a somewhat haphazard fashion, hoping like hell it all comes together correctly at the end. Cowboy is also used to refer to a surgeon who perhaps doesn't have the best judgment—someone who operates first and asks questions later."

Unlike romantic notions of the Wild West cowboy, when the term is used in medicine, it's an insult.

"To me, a cowboy is the worst thing you can be called," says Dr. Erin Sullivan, a newly graduated physician from Ireland's University of Limerick who returned to her native Canada in July 2013 to do a residency in rural family medicine in Saskatchewan.

One ER nurse knows all about medical cowboys. She remembers working with a doctor who she called a cowboy because he did invasive procedures—usually without local anesthetic and definitely without warning. "We had a kid who came in with an abscess on his neck," the nurse recalls. "The kid was sitting on the mom's lap and the doctor had a scalpel in his hand. And he just said, 'Look, at your mom.' The kid turned and he literally plunged the scalpel right in the neck. The kid obviously flipped out."

When the nurse reproached the doctor later that day, he said the alternative was to restrain the child by wrapping him in a blanket and pinning him to the stretcher. The possibility of giving pain relievers and sedation by intravenous drip or at least injecting the skin over the abscess with local anesthetic had obviously not occurred to the doctor. "Those people I find are the most frightening to work with," she says.

Surgical resident Dr. Christopher Kinsella has a reflective take on cowboys. He defines a cowboy as a surgeon undertaking a risky operation for marginal benefit in which the patient bears the consequences. "In one sense, it's my risk. But if I fail, the person who suffers is you," says Kinsella. "If you're making those types of decisions on behalf of your patients, it's almost always inappropriate. And that's what makes you a cowboy."

I find Kinsella's take startling; for a young surgeon to accuse colleagues of operating with reckless abandon is unusual.

////////

The common slang term for orthopedic surgeons is *orthopods*. It doesn't sound like an insult to me, but it does to them.

The term "doesn't go over well with orthopedic surgeons," says Peter Kussin. What makes it an insult is its similarity to the word *anthropoid*—animals in a category that includes apes and gorillas. It suggests that orthopedic surgeons are a step behind in evolutionary terms. In hospital corridors, Kussin says, orthopedic surgeons are often referred to by unflatteringly as knuckle scrapers and knuckle draggers.

Back inside the anesthesia residents' lounge at one of the top hospitals in America, a first-year resident told me about a cartoon skit on YouTube called "Orthopedia vs. Anesthesia" in which an orthopedic surgeon proposes to fix a broken bone on a dead patient. The message is clear: orthopedic surgeons like to operate so much it clouds their judgment.

"I feel bad for picking on the orthopedic surgeons, but oftentimes you'll get these 90- or 100-year-old patients who need a hip pinning," says a third-year anesthesiology resident. "And they've got 100 co-morbidities and [take] 1,000 medications. These patients couldn't tell you their own name, much less the date or the time."

More and more, the job of caring for the non-orthopedic medical needs of such frail elderly patients goes to specialists in internal medicine, says a resident in internal medicine. Once when he was on call, he was asked to see an elderly woman just back from the operating room, where an orthopedic surgeon had fixed her broken hip. That night, she was agitated and so the orthopedic surgeon ordered an injection of five milligrams of haloperidol, an antipsychotic drug used frequently in hospitals to sedate disruptive and violent patients.

"You come to see the patient in the morning and they're completely snowed and the tone in their muscles is completely stiff because of the medications," says the resident. "You try and find the surgeon [for an explanation] but they're in the operating room, so you can't talk to them."

FOOBA, which stands for "found on ortho barely alive," describes this situation. Some doctors call it FDOOBA for "found down on ortho barely alive."

"There's this basic perception that orthopedic surgeons are very good technicians at fixing bones and doing the procedures that they do," says Dr. Zubin Damania. "But other than that, they know not a lick of medicine." Damania's duties as a hospitalist include handling the medical stuff (as he calls it) that his orthopedic colleagues fail to do. "A lot of times you'll get a call and the patient is barely alive [on the orthopedic ward] because they've already screwed things up so much that by the time you stumble onto the case, you're basically trying to undo all these horrible things done by neglect."

An experienced internist I know says he's seen many patients in orthopedic wards who have been put into heart failure because their surgeons gave them too much IV fluids, causing shortness of breath. Then they call on my colleague to save the patient. "It's always the same thing," says the internist. "They don't even know that they caused it."

This insult has more than a grain of truth. More and more hospitals have hired hospitalists like Damania to manage the non-surgical issues that patients on orthopedic wards face—so they don't die after they survive surgery.

In fairness, I asked an orthopedic surgery resident who is training at one of the top hospitals in America if FOOBA has any truth to it. "I think some of it's deserved," said the resident. "It seems like we're better off fixing bones."

On the other hand, the resident says, you should hear what orthopedic surgeons have to say about the diagnostic skill of their internal medicine colleagues. "They don't know how to do any kind of muscle-skeletal exam whatsoever," the resident says. "They know that somebody's knee hurts, so they get a consult in orthopedics."

He and other residents have a name for that kind of referral. They call it a garbage consult.

Dr. Peter Kussin says it's not simply a case of one specialty not knowing how to diagnose clinical problems that fall under another specialty. He says there's a deeper problem—doing a superficial assessment of the patient instead of keeping close tabs. There's even a slang term for that: LGFD, which stands for "looks good from door."

"That would be probably the most derogatory thing I would say about a physician, because to me that's just totally a professional lapse of their responsibilities," says Kussin.

///////

Bone surgeons may not have a great reputation for looking after the non-orthopedic medical needs of their patients. But at least they're appreciated for their judgment and skill in the operating room. The same is not necessarily said of specialists in obstetrics and gynecology.

A third-year resident at one of America's top hospitals told me a story that calls into question the awareness—if not the competence—of a resident in obstetrics and gynecology.

"We do about 95 to 99 percent of our Caesarean sections under spinal anesthesia and so, of course, the patient is awake," says the resident. "In May of my first year of residency, [I was] working with an upper-level OBGYN resident who was having trouble closing the incision at the end of a Caesarean section. The resident kind of looked at me and said, 'Is there anything we can do about the patient's breathing? It's kind of tough to close the wound. Can we turn the ventilator off?'"

There was no ventilator to shut off because the patient wasn't on a ventilator. The anesthesiology resident tells me he had performed a spinal block—which meant the patient wasn't under a general anesthetic, was breathing on her own and was awake (and listening in).

"Ma'am, could you hold your breath?" the anesthesiology resident asked the woman.

"It was just obvious that the resident had no idea what was going on, which was kind of astonishing. I wish that was the only story I had."

///////

Surgical cowboys are seen as health care's unthinking doers. Internists—non-surgical specialists who are experts in diseases such as diabetes, heart failure and high blood pressure—are polar opposites: obsessive thinkers who don't do much of anything. What do we call doctors like that? We call them fleas.

Dr. Ryan Madanick, a gastroenterologist, remembers the first time he was called a flea was when he was a resident in internal medicine. A resident in surgery "looked at me and called me a fucking flea," Madanick recalls. "Then she explained that *flea* stands for 'fucking little esoteric asshole.' Surgeons don't think like we do. They're not as smart as us. Therefore, it's actually a compliment. We're smarter than they are," says Madanick.

Not everyone believes the term *flea* comes from the acronym Madanick learned.

"I like the idea that the last thing that leaves a dead body are fleas," says Kussin. "To me, that's the most poetic." He says he's heard but doesn't much like the idea that the term comes from comparing the stethoscopes internal medicine doctors wear to flea collars. "I find that pedestrian." Another possible origin "is that there are more internal medicine people on rounds than fleas on a dog."

One word that does ring true in the acronym for Kussin is *esoteric*. Internists are nothing if not that. "It is the ultimate disrespect for our sort of nattering around, never making decisions and arguing about esoterica in the face of someone who's dying while not recognizing that they're dying."

Take dying of a gunshot wound, for example, says Kussin. "We would look at a gunshot wound and say, 'That's acute lead poisoning. Get a lead level.' The surgeons would make fun of us for that."

That's the punchline to a joke; but is there any truth to the critique? "Of course," says Kussin. "I think surgeons properly identify us as being focused on minutiae."

But somebody has to do that. There's a saying in medicine: "Common things occur commonly." Rare diagnoses do not come quickly to my brain. But they do to internists. They revel in them. They even have a nickname for rare diagnoses; they call them zebras.

I was struck by the fact that Ryan Madanick immediately saw a compliment buried in a sandbox insult. At least *cowboy* conjures up a romantic image in our culture; not so the flea. But that doesn't bother Peter Kussin. "I wear it pretty proudly," he says.

Still, let's not forget that to a non-internist, being called a flea is an insult. A veteran ER physician told me she thinks of the word *flea* whenever she's desperate to get the internist on call to accept a referral but the internist is giving her a hard time. "Whenever that happens, the internist is asking some picky little question or asking if I have considered some obscure diagnosis," says the ER physician. "Seriously, when I look at how busy my emergency room is, and I get that treatment, that's when I know I'm dealing with a flea."

///////

In modern medical culture, specialists are seen as smart overachievers, while generalists such as family docs and ER physicians are seen as less intelligent and less ambitious. It's an attitude that is reflected in everything from the status accorded the physicians to the money they make.

"The nickname internal medicine uses for emergency room physician is *triage monkey* or *glorified triage nurse*," says Dr. Nathan Stall. "I've heard that time and time again."

Triage—which comes from the French verb *trier*, which means to sort or to sift—is the process of deciding which patients go first based on the gravity of their condition. When you come to the ER with an illness or an injury, the triage nurse is the first person you see. Using a combination of rules or algorithms, plus intuition honed by years of experience, the triage nurse figures out when it's your turn. Get it wrong—for example, leave a woman with an ectopic, or tubal, pregnancy sitting too long in the waiting room—and there's a good chance the patient will go into shock and die.

Triage nurses also have to field incessant questions and complaints from patients and aggressive family members wondering when it's their turn. You could not pay me enough to do their job.

Calling me a triage nurse trivializes what triage nurses do shift in and shift out—which is to save our bacon by making sure ER physicians see patients in time to save them. And the term trivializes what I do as an ER doctor—by suggesting I assess patients too quickly and too superficially.

An ER colleague of mine who works in Ottawa told me about

a similar slang term that describes ER physicians. "A *referologist* is the slang term that we use for an ER colleague who can't make a decision and likes to refer everybody," says the resident. "It tends to be used more by the consultants about us, but we use it amongst ourselves as well."

Both *referologist* and *triage monkey* suggest that specialists are smarter than ER physicians and family doctors—a belief reinforced by professors in med school. Dr. Jason Quinn remembers first hearing it when he went to the University of Western Ontario in London, Ontario. "Every lecture is started and ended with the family physician screwing up and the specialist riding to the rescue," says Quinn.

Now a psychiatrist in training, Quinn says fellow residents trade tips on which ER doctors are quick to refer patients with apparent psychiatric problems. "Doctor so-and-so is on duty in the emergency department," says Quinn. "That means we're going to get a lot of bad referrals."

Like Quinn, Stall says residents in internal medicine trade the same intelligence. "If this guy's on tonight, you can expect some shitty consults," says Stall.

Loose talk like that is dangerous to hospital culture. Casual disparaging of a colleague to others is considered a breach of professional ethics; more than that, it's a violation of the code of just getting along.

My research for this book has given me an unprecedented opportunity to hear other specialists complain not just about one another but about ER physicians like me. Internists think we order too many tests, like CT scans, and IV antibiotics without good reason. They're probably right. Still, we work under time pressure that would frankly make most internists panic. We're supposed to know a little bit about every field of medicine. We never know who or what kind of problem is coming through the sliding doors next.

Like every other physician I know, we hate being second-guessed by a surgeon or an internist. By their nature, physicians love to point out the clinical shortcomings of their colleagues. Having a good story to tell at the expense of an ER physician more than makes up for any extra work.

It may be verboten for surgeons or internists to rail against ER doctors openly. But there's one exception. It's perfectly acceptable to talk down another specialty to try to prevent a colleague from changing career paths.

An ER colleague of mine discovered that while doing a residency in ear, nose and throat (ENT), when she told her mentors she wanted to switch training positions and become an ER physician. "'Why would you want to be a triage doctor?'" she recalls them asking her. "To be honest, I was hurt by it at the time. I do think that ER physicians treat and discharge many patients who never see the specialist. They forget that. The bigger picture is that we actually save them a lot of unnecessary referrals."

//////

You may be getting the false impression that, in the us-versus-them world of hospital medicine, an honour code prevents members of a specialty from making fun of one another. That's not true. Dr. Chris Kinsella is quite happy to rant about the cowboys among his surgical colleagues. ER doctors complain about each other in the same way.

A fellow ER physician once told me about a colleague who was known as a money-grubber. He worked too quickly for his own competence and saw double the number of patients as the second-fastest doctor. His histories and physicals were superficial. Despite his high-volume practice, he had an uncanny knack for leaving on time. By comparison, most of my colleagues and I see far fewer patients—which means we get paid much less—yet stay an hour or two beyond the official finish time of our shifts to tie off loose ends.

How did he do it? By handing over patients who had been worked up incompletely to the ER doctor on the next shift. Every once in a while, tucked away among the six or seven patients he had left for the next ER doc to finish up was a patient who contained what an ER colleague who works in another province calls a hidden bomb —a life-threatening medical problem the doctor doing the hand-over failed to notice and to warn colleagues about. I call my friend's money-grubbing colleague the Bomb-maker.

Handing over patients is one of the riskiest things ER physicians do because the second ER doctor seldom has time to retake the history. If the first doctor got it wrong, the patient may be doomed.

Another colleague recalls working a morning shift in which he was handed the mother of hidden bombs. The patient had chest pain, and the doctor doing the handover said the patient could go home after a blood test ruled out a heart attack. No biggie. The night doctor went home, and the colleague decided to see the patient himself.

"I went in and he was literally on death's door," he says. "He had an aortic dissection."

An aortic dissection is the hydrogen bomb of hidden ordnance. It's a life-threatening condition caused by a tear in the inner wall of the aorta, the big artery that comes off the heart and sweeps around and through the chest and into the abdomen. Dissections that rupture have an 80 percent mortality rate.

In 2009, famed Canadian soprano Measha Brueggergosman nearly joined the list. She had chest pain and went to St. Joseph's Hospital in the west end of downtown Toronto, where she was seen by doctors and sent home. Fortunately, she called her family doctor, who told the opera singer to go another hospital, where the correct diagnosis was made in time to save her life.

My colleague's patient likewise made it. "That was a hidden bomb that was defused in time," he says.

Those of us who have bomb-maker stories to tell should not get sanctimonious. Every ER physician has left a bomb or two behind, including me. It's just that when you're handed over a bomb that goes off, a patient can get really sick or die. If not blamed for what happened, at the very least you get sucked into a maelstrom of complaints and litigation.

And you learn never to trust that colleague at handover again.

///////

When doctors use slang to talk about each other, it's as likely to be about their attitude as about their competence.

As a neurologist, Dr. Grumpy has referred many patients to neurosurgeons to do everything from clipping aneurysms to removing brain tumours. His take on them is refreshingly candid: "I do think that they are good doctors with just crappy personalities." He cares more about neurosurgeons' competence than their attitude. "If my patient needs surgery," he says, "I really don't care whether or not you're a jackass."

It's not surprising that Dr. Grumpy doesn't care whether the neurosurgeons he works with are jackasses. Although he refers patients to them, he doesn't have to work alongside them in a high-risk environment like the operating room. That's the job of the anesthesiologists. They have strong opinions plus some graphic slang they use to describe the personalities of their surgical colleagues.

"I can only speak from my experience, but some of the orthopedic surgeons can be difficult," says the first-year anesthesiology resident at one of America's top hospitals. "Some of the general surgeons can be difficult. Some of the transplant surgeons can be difficult."

A colleague of his who is in the third year of anesthesiology residency at the same hospital has a slightly different take. "Unequivocally, after [my] three years of training, the neurosurgeons and the cardiothoracic surgeons are the most difficult to work with."

Volumes have been written about difficult physicians, of whom many are surgeons. But even cancer specialists make the list. Dr. Grumpy remembers attending a cancer conference in the U.S. several years ago at which experts in radiation and chemotherapy met to discuss the best course of treatment for patients with cancer. An argument broke out at the podium between a radiation oncologist and a chemotherapy guru. "It just kept escalating," Dr. Grumpy recalls. "When one had a turn to present, the other kept interrupting him or making snide remarks. The argument became increasingly heated. At some point, they got up and began pushing each other and then began punching and had to be separated."

When I was a med student, it was common knowledge that a well-known and highly respected surgeon was infamous for throwing scalpels at hapless assistants in the OR. But that was thirty years go. It would be nice to think doctors have evolved since then. But a 2004 survey published in the journal *Physician Executive* found a staggering 95 percent of hospital and clinic executives have to deal with disruptive physicians as a regular part of their jobs. A 2011 survey for the American College of Physician Executives found twenty-seven of nearly 850 physicians had exhibited disruptive behaviour at least once in their career.

There are several reasons physicians have been too slow to clean up their act. Ironically, at the top of the list is the fact that colleagues tend to admire them. In a 2009 article published in the *Journal of Medical Regulation*, psychiatrist Dr. Norman Reynolds pointed out that difficult doctors are thought of as highly skilled, well-read, intelligent, articulate, hardworking, confident and persevering. Those characteristics kind of make up for arrogant, intimidating, inflexible, self-centred and unempathetic, don't you think?

Dr. Thomas Krizek, a surgeon, wrote a scathing account of bad behaviour by surgical colleagues it was published in 2002 in the *Journal of the American College of Surgeons*. In it, Krizek argued that students and residents tolerate abusive surgeons—bad role models though they may be—because they see them as entertaining and charismatic.

"Students and residents are often in awe, albeit terrified at the same time," wrote Krizek. "This behaviour may be interpreted by residents as reflecting the behaviour of 'champions' against the establishment; it is no wonder that residents wish to emulate their behaviour."

I think that the hierarchical structure of hospital medicine tends to attract abusive physicians. Not surprisingly, nurses and residents—who are well below attending physicians in the hospital food chain—bear the brunt of abuse by attending physicians.

The 1993 article in *Social Science & Medicine* by Robert Coombs and his co-authors referred to an attending physician who attacks and shreds medical trainees without provocation as a "shark." and residents referred to attending rounds as "offending rounds."

A 2011 article by Barbara Barzansky and Sylvia Etzel in the *Journal of the American Medical Association* says the percentage of women in medical schools rose from 36 percent in 1990 to more than 48 percent 20 years later.

It has long been hoped—if not believed fervently—that women physicians are less likely to be disruptive than their male counterparts. But a 2013 story in the *Washington Post* puts paid to that. Reporter Sandra Boodman wrote about how a surgeon in the midst of a complex operation reacted when a technician handed her a device that didn't work properly: "Furious that she couldn't use it, the surgeon slammed it down, accidentally breaking the technician's finger."

The 2011 survey for the American College of Physician

Executives found that 27 percent of male physicians had been disruptive—and so had 23 percent of their female counterparts. The presence of women physicians in growing numbers may reduce the number of difficult colleagues as well as disruptive acts, but not nearly as much as some have hoped.

An unfortunate byproduct of the emergence of women in traditionally male areas of medicine (general surgery, orthopedics and neurosurgery) is abusive behaviour toward female trainees. In his article, Krizek gave a chilling example: a senior surgeon waved a suction device in the face of a female medical student and announced that "he was going to stick the sucker so far up her ass that it would suck out her brains, if she had any."

Krizek's article was published back in 2002. But abuse and disrespect towards women are apparently alive and well today. "We will talk about residents 'having hypervaginosis,'" says a former senior resident in general surgery. *Hypervaginosis* is pure slang. Vaginosis is a clinical term for an infection of the vagina. The prefix *hyper-* means "excessive." I asked my informant to define hypervaginosis. "Forgive me, but they're a big pussy," he replied.

I asked him what would it take for a resident to get a reputation for hypervaginosis.

"Complaining, [especially] to someone outside the hierarchy or chain of command," said the young doctor. "We have a resident who all of us have had issues with because she frequently complains about something to the program director rather than her senior resident or chief resident or someone basically in that chain. We like to think of ourselves as being very hierarchical; even as a chief resident, I would very seldom go to the chairman of the department with a problem.

"Going outside of that gives you a reputation as whining, as being very complaining, as having a lot to complain about and not respecting that some things aren't badness. Not expecting that, you are going to have some problems because it's residency and it's surgery and it can be very difficult."

I asked who came up with the term *hypervaginosis.*

"I have no idea," he said. The former chief resident said he did his medical school at a college in another state. He was sure he had not heard *hypervaginosis* until he started his residency in general surgery.

And what does author Dr. Stephen Bergman think about the slang term and its meaning? "I think that's despicable," he says. "It's saying you're whining because you're a woman. You know, a pussy is a sort of weak, whining woman. I'll put it this way. From all my years in the pre-women's movement and the women's movement, I have seen the tremendous destruction that kind of shit does. You just don't do that. We would never have done that. Ever."

Disruptive or abusive behaviour has a serious effect on hospital culture. Norman Reynolds wrote that it "demoralizes members of the hospital staff, leads to lawsuits by co-workers, and can create a hostile work environment."

It also affects the safety of patients. The 2008 Sentinel Event Alert by the Joint Commission said: "Intimidating and disruptive behaviors can foster medical errors, contribute to poor patient satisfaction and to preventable adverse outcomes, increase the cost of care, and cause qualified clinicians, administrators and managers to seek new positions in more professional environments." Beginning in January 2009, the Joint Commission required hospitals to develop zero tolerance for such behaviors.

In his article, Dr. Norman Reynolds concluded that preventing disruptive behaviour is better than having to deal with it on the job. He recommended screening job seekers for prior unprofessional behaviour. More controversially, he explored the possibility of looking for worrisome patterns in applicants to medical school.

Good luck with that. It's easy to make new rules to discourage disruptive doctors; much harder to change the culture that bred them. It turns out that disruptive doctors often bring lots of paying patients into the hospital. The 2008 Sentinel Event Alert said that hospital staff perceive that revenue-generating doctors are "let off the hook" for bad behaviour; nearly 40 percent of physician executives surveyed in 2004 agreed that "physicians in my organization who generate high amounts of revenue are treated more leniently when it comes to behaviour problems than those who bring in less revenue."

You'll know the problem is ebbing when doctors and nurses stop inventing slang to talk down their colleagues. So far, that hasn't happened.

///////

With slang terms like *cowboy* and *flea*, it's easy to get the sense that surgeons, internists, ER doctors and everyone else have nothing in common. Envy and jealousy over money, power and influence are the things that divide us. Still, if there's one thing that binds us together, it's those powerful, life-changing traumatic occurrences to which each of us must bear witness. As you'll see, we have slang for those too.

CHAPTER THIRTEEN

Horrendomas

O ne of the first bits of argot I learned when I was a resident is the made-up word *horrendoma*. Take *horrendous* and tack on *-oma*, the medical suffix for tumour. Pseudodictionary.com defines a horrendoma as "denoting an unusually bad or complicated medical condition."

Every profession, every job, every business has a slang word for those times when everything goes wrong. Many call it a snafu, the sarcastic military expression that means "situation normal: all fucked up." The fact that your life might be on the line adds more than a bit of tension to the mix—and makes the stories my colleagues share all the more spine-tingling.

Dr. Jay Ross, an anesthesiologist, has another name for horrendoma. "When there is an emergency happening and everything seems to be spinning a little out of control, and there's not really a sense of what's going on, we call it a clusterfuck."

The phrase comes from the old adage that anesthesiology is "98 percent boredom and 2 percent sheer terror." Anesthesiologists are responsible not only for delivering anesthesia in the operating room but also for keeping patients safe during surgery. The hallmark of that job is what we call securing the airway. That means intubating (placing an endotracheal tube past the larynx and into the trachea), followed by putting the patient on a ventilator. Any number of obstacles—arthritic neck, congenitally tiny jaw, large tongue, floppy uvula, stiff epiglottis, to name a few—can stand in the anesthesiologist's way.

Clusterfuck is a reminder that no matter how well they plan their work, one day a patient will arrive whose airway puts all of the anesthesiologist's training to the test. That's what happened to Jay Ross during a night on call as a staff anesthesiologist.

Ross was called in the middle of the night to the intensive care unit for a patient with bleeding esophageal varices, extremely dilated veins in the lower part of the esophagus. These are most commonly associated with cirrhosis of the liver. The problem with varices is that they can cause massive bleeding in the esophagus, which can cause the patient to go into shock. I've seen a patient nearly bleed to death in minutes. That's bad enough, but the bleeding can be so brisk that it blocks the airway and threatens to suffocate the patient. Ross was called to the ICU that night to secure the man's airway because the ICU doctors hadn't been able to.

"They couldn't intubate this bleeding person, and now they were calling me," says Ross. When he opened the patient's mouth, all he saw was blood pouring out like a fountain.

"Oh my god, this guy was just spewing blood nonstop," Ross recalls. "I was having a hard time seeing the vocal cords so I could pass an endotracheal tube to protect his airway. I remember trying every trick in the book. I even got someone to press down on the chest and I looked for the air bubbles through the blood to try to put the tube in."

Ross tried one assistive device after another—every toy, as he called them, available to him. Each failed, and the patient's throat kept filling up with blood. Eventually, Ross was able to provide the patient with some oxygen and buy time for a final attempt to save him by using a device called a laryngeal mask airway.

"I know we were certainly pushing blood into his lungs, but there was no choice," says Ross, who summoned a surgeon to make a hole in the middle of the patient's trachea called a cricothyroidotomy and pass a breathing tube through the hole. "You could almost feel this audible sigh. You could see the lungs rising. To give credit to the surgeon, I didn't secure the airway, the surgeon did."

Unfortunately, it was all for naught. The patient continued to bleed and went into irreversible shock; he died several hours later in the ICU. "Coming back later and hearing that he'd died was just frustrating," says Ross. "You put all this energy into trying to save this person's life, and it was all for naught. Really."

What happened to Ross was a clusterfuck because anything that could go wrong did.

An ear, nose and throat (ENT) surgeon who does facial plastic surgery in the Pacific Northwest calls that sort of thing a Humpty Dumpty for the nursery rhyme guy they couldn't put together again. He remembers the first time he heard the phrase. "It was actually an orthopedic surgery and I was an intern," says the ENT surgeon. "It was a pelvic fracture. When they are simple, you just put one plate or one rod through the bone. When you have some high-velocity, high-energy impact, the bones will just shatter. When I got woken up to go to the operating room, my senior resident said, 'We've got a Humpty Dumpty we have to go fix.' I remember that vividly, because I thought it was kind of smart and not so derogatory. It just kind of illustrated to me what we had to go do. There was a goal of rehabilitation there. That's why I don't get turned off by that phrase."

Every physician I know has a horrendoma memory or two that keep him or her awake at night. If you have lots of them, your colleagues might begin to refer to you as a black cloud or a shit magnet.

But here's the thing. As physicians, none of this is supposed to affect us. And we have a venerable physician named Sir William Osler to thank for that. Osler, one of the founders of modern medicine, first made a name for himself at McGill University in Montreal before heading to the United States. At The Johns Hopkins Hospital in Baltimore, Maryland, Osler became that pre-eminent institution's first professor of medicine—one of the four founding professors of the hospital. Osler created the first residency-training program for graduate physicians.

Among Osler's lasting contributions is a legacy of essays intended to impart his wisdom to the physicians of tomorrow. *Aequanimitas* is Osler's most famous essay; it admonishes MDs to maintain an attitude of unflappability that he referred to as "imperturbability."

Wrote Osler: "Imperturbability means coolness and presence of mind under all circumstances, calmness amid storm, clearness of judgment in moments of grave peril, immobility, impassiveness, or, to use an old and expressive word, *phlegm*.... Even under the most serious circumstances, the physician or surgeon who ... shows in his face the slightest alteration, expressive of anxiety or fear, has not his medullary centres under the highest control, and is liable to disaster at any moment."

Simply put, Osler admonished generations of physicians—including me—never to let patients and their families see us sweat. Today, we call it detachment. But the concept is the same. "There is a long-standing tension in the physician's role," Dr. Jodi Halpern, a psychiatrist and philosopher, wrote in an article published in 2003 in the *Journal of General Internal Medicine*. "On the one hand, doctors strive for detachment to reliably care for all patients, regardless of their personal feelings. Yet patients want genuine empathy from doctors, and doctors want to provide it."

Finding the balance between emotional detachment and concern for the patient is the great challenge of modern medicine. Osler lived at a time when disease was the main cause of death, and death was accepted as part of life, even in infancy and childbirth. Today, people are more likely to die in violent circumstances—everything from horrific car crashes to child abuse; these leave their mark on the survivors and on the healers. Such experiences are daily occurrences for modern physicians and surgeons. You would have to be a fool to think they leave no emotional scars.

I strongly doubt Sir William Osler used, much less invented, medical slang to describe the sad and horrible things that happen to patients that he witnessed as part of his job. But we do. And I would argue that in a perverse, unintended sort of way, we have Osler to thank for it.

My first horrendoma happened when I was asked for the first time to pronounce a person dead in the ER—a story I told in my book *The Night Shift*. A woman had left the psychiatric hospital where she was a patient, walked to the nearest subway station, and leaped in front of an approaching train.

As I approached her body, I realized in horror that her face was pointing at the ceiling, yet her torso was pointing down toward the floor. The speeding subway train had decapitated the woman; the paramedics had arranged her head above her neck to make her appear more human—but they had ignored a rather important anatomical detail.

I kept my Oslerian composure long enough to complete the formalities. It was only after I left the room and retreated to the emergency physicians' office that I could allow myself a moment to fall to my knees—giddy, nauseous and sick at heart from the experience. It was weeks before I could close my eyes without seeing the woman's absurdly placid face.

For nearly twenty years, I was angry with the paramedics who had me pronounce the woman without pulling me aside and telling me what I was about to witness. But, more recently, I began to feel bad for *them*. Did anybody warn them what they would find when they retrieved her body from the tracks?

Morgan Jones Phillips, one of the most passionate and articulate paramedics I've ever met, knows more about such horrendous incidents than I would ever want to know.

"How many jumpers have I done?" Phillips asks. "I've probably done ten in eight years. We have something called Code Five; it means that they're obviously dead in a way that means you should not try to help them."

Phillips says Code Five means the paramedics do not have to begin life-saving procedures such as CPR and defibrillation. It usually has one of several outcomes—each a horrendoma. There may be a body with no pulse to feel and obvious signs of death such as rigor mortis, dependent lividity (a blue or purple discoloration in the body where blood has settled), or a rotting appearance and smell of putrefaction. The body may be burned beyond recognition.

A Code Five also refers to instances that are almost too horrific to describe. The body might be split in two across the torso. Or, like the woman I pronounced dead in the ER, the victim may have been decapitated. Phillips remembers a victim like that—a story he describes as an Ugly Code Five.

"He was actually quite a *thoughtful* guy," Phillips says with a tinge of detached sarcasm, marvelling at the pains the jumper took not to be an inconvenience. "He had gone into the subway at the end of the night, at closing time. He hid at the end of the platform and waited for the night car that drives through the stations to collect the garbage. Just before the car entered the station, he jumped down off the platform, stuck his head out and rested his neck across the tracks, and the train ran over his head.

"In situations like that, the patient is the poor guy who's driving the garbage car. The driver shouldn't, but he's going to feel like he's killed him and is going to have to deal with that. In that situation, *he* becomes our patient."

For paramedics like Phillips, the most disturbing on-the-job memories are those in which the victim—while undeniably dead—*looks* unharmed. Such victims do not meet the strict criteria for a Code Five, which means paramedics must attempt to rescue them, even though it's obvious they are dead. Phillips recalls one such man, also a subway suicide.

"We had to do everything, but he was under a subway train," Phillips recalls. "My partner and I crawled under the car, feeling terrified. Then we got him out from under it. And when we tried to move him, it was obvious that every bone was broken. He wasn't even bleeding. We picked him up by the arms and legs, but there were no bones to speak of at all. Everything was just sort of crushed."

Despite the fact the man did not meet the tight requirements of a Code Five, Phillips said he and his partner contacted authorities and received permission to pronounce the man dead in the field. To Phillips, the most disturbing part of the story was that the man appeared well enough to get up and walk away, despite the horrific way he'd met his death.

How paramedics like Phillips cope with horrendomas like these is a matter of great concern. Studies have shown that paramedics have a much higher prevalence of post-traumatic stress disorder (PTSD) than the general population. PTSD is a severe anxiety disorder that sometimes occurs following a psychological trauma. The trauma can be a threat to your own life or your witnessing of a threat to someone else's life. It can lead to chronic anxiety, depression, substance abuse, marital breakup, loss of employment and suicide. Although Emergency Medicine Services have implemented programs aimed at early recognition and treatment for paramedics, the culture of paramedicine often promotes a pattern of denial among working paramedics—perhaps yet another of Osler's legacies.

Some paramedics like to talk about traumatic calls, but most, like Phillips, prefer to keep those memories to themselves.

"I'm sort of a suppress-and-move-on kind of guy," he says. "I'm not saying it's healthy or correct, but I don't even really talk to my wife about the bad calls."

///////

You never hear physicians talking about PTSD unless it's about a patient with the problem. The thing is, we're just as susceptible, yet we don't believe it can happen to us. But consider this: what surgeons and ER docs see every day would probably cause PTSD in most people. Unlike paramedics, doctors like me seldom have to scoop up dead bodies. But we do have our moments when we encounter cadavers as part of our medical studies and later as part of our work. And, earlier in the history of medical education, dissecting a cadaver in anatomy class and the first autopsy were often made into highly ritualized experiences for budding physicians.

One woman who knows a great deal about medical education is Dr. Renee Fox, one of the pioneers of medical sociology. In the 1950s, Fox was associated with the "medical school project," a long-term study of the sociology of the medical education of students at Columbia University in New York City. As part of her four-year research in the field, Fox observed second-year medical students at Columbia as they attended their first autopsies as part of a course in general pathology.

In her essay "The Autopsy: Its Place in the Attitude-Learning of Second-Year Medical Students" (first published in 1979), Fox wrote that the autopsy was regarded by students as one of the "landmark" or "milestone" experiences of their training in medical school. She emphasized that the experience was not simply about advancing the students' intellectual development; but that the students "also describe participation in an autopsy as 'an emotionally important experience . . . one of the hurdles you have to get over along the way to becoming a doctor.'"

Fox was struck most by the notion that the ritual of the first autopsy helps teach budding physicians how to demonstrate "detached concern," a process by which "students gradually learn to combine the counter attitudes of detachment and concern to attain the balance between objectivity and empathy expected of mature physicians in the various kinds of professional situations they encounter."

She emphasized the ritualistic aspect of the experience of the first autopsy as helping to prepare students to develop a sense of detached concern. The first autopsy itself was invested with a sense of occasion in which the students experienced a number of firsts—the first time being on call and literally waiting for a patient to die, and the first time students don scrub suits.

Fox examined an aspect of the culture of modern medicine— first articulated by Osler—that continues to this day: peer pressure to deny the emotional impact of such experiences. "Students share the unspoken conviction that 'admitting you had qualms about the autopsy' or that 'it made you feel queasy' is not in keeping with standards of professional objectivity," Fox wrote. She also noted that the students themselves limited the extent to which they discussed the autopsy among themselves so as to "avert an excessively emotional response to it."

Fox captured clearly the dilemma faced by the students—and, I would argue, physicians like me; that is, how to look at the work we do objectively while still being able to feel things emotionally.

Fox's study of medical students predates my own experience by a quarter of a century. In my first year of medical school, my classmate Eric Deigan (now an OBGYN in North Carolina) and I dissected a cadaver as part of our anatomy class. I recall that there were six to eight cadavers in each seminar room arranged in two rows of three or four each. For an entire semester, we dissected parts of the cadavers to illustrate what we had learned in the lecture hall.

I remember the strong smell of formaldehyde, the preservative used to keep the bodies from rotting. It filled my nostrils and so covered my hands that it would take hours after each dissection to regain my appetite. Most of the time, I was in awe of the man who donated his body so that I could learn about human anatomy.

The first incision my partner and I made into the cadaver's body made me feel physically sick. To ease my squeamishness, I remember making lots of jokes about it. I nicknamed my cadaver Ernest so that if anyone outside of medicine asked how I spent my time, I could reply: "I'm working in dead Ernest."

In her research from the 1950s, Fox noted that students made jokes about the dissection.

"Gallows humor flourished in the anatomy laboratory, where the students were literally faced with cutting into dead human persons," said Fox in an interview. "That was their first encounter with death in that rather special form."

However, Fox said, there were occasions while dissecting cadavers when the gallows humour was put away. "I was also struck by the fact that they didn't make jokes during the particular high emotional points in the dissection, which were not only working on the genitalia of the cadaver, but even more so on the hands and on the face, where the humanness of the body lying on the table asserted itself."

For me, the most difficult moment came the day Eric and I dissected our cadaver's face. As we cut away the layers of skin and fascia underneath, the cadaver lost its humanness. When I went home that day, I looked at myself in the mirror and realized that what separated me from him were three layers of cells—the thickness of which is roughly the diameter of a pin.

The connection to a recently living human being—what Morgan Jones Phillips alluded to when he described the body of the man that he and his partner lifted from the subway tracks—is what connects us to the cadaver in the anatomy class and the autopsy room.

Fox concluded that the first autopsy plays an important role in medical students' development of detached concern for patients. But the autopsy rate in the U.S. has been in steep decline since 1972. In 2011, the Centers for Disease Control's National Center for Health Statistics reported that the percentage of deaths for which autopsies were performed dropped by more than 50 percent—from 19.3 percent in 1972 to just 8.5 percent a quarter of a century later. Other countries—including Canada, Australia and Denmark—have also seen sharp declines in autopsy rates.

Several reasons account for this. In the U.S., Medicaid and health insurers don't pay for autopsies. In 1971, the Joint Commission dropped its requirement that hospitals have an autopsy rate of 20 to 25 percent of the deaths that occur in them. Some have suggested that doctors are less likely to ask the family to agree to an autopsy out of the belief that MRIs and other modern diagnostic imaging techniques obviate their need. Studies have suggested physicians are reluctant to ask for autopsies for fear of triggering a lawsuit. Others believe doctors are trying to respect religions and cultures that prohibit or frown on autopsies.

I think physicians no longer ask for autopsies because they no longer think they're worthwhile. Likewise, I suspect that physicians no longer believe in the carefully crafted sense of detached concern nurtured in medical students as described by Renee Fox and other medical sociologists.

Whatever the reason, without the ritualistic structure of the autopsy as a milestone experience, it's entirely possible that medical students might be learning to be less *detached* and more *concerned* about their patients—a cause for celebration.

////////

All doctors struggle to find the balance between detachment and emotional openness; for surgeons, the sweet spot is by far the trickiest. My surgical colleagues spend years developing the technical skill and gathering the experience necessary to put patients under the knife safely.

"For me, the conduct of an operation is largely about focus and discipline," says Dr. Marcus Burnstein, a colorectal surgeon at St. Michael's Hospital in Toronto. "The focus is on the steps of the operation, and the discipline is to ensure that every step is completed without shortcuts or compromises."

The technical demands of surgery are obvious. You need unparalleled manual dexterity, stamina and the ability to go patiently through a series of complex steps in order. It also helps if you have prodigious attention to visual detail.

The thing I find many surgeons fail to appreciate is that an operation is a form of controlled violence on the patient. If surgeons thought about what they do to patients on a daily basis, I suspect many wouldn't do it. Even the most successful surgery causes severe (albeit manageable) pain. For patients relieved of their condition, post-operative pain is bearable—but not so much when the surgery results in complications or worse.

"You asked if emotional detachment is necessary, and for me I think the answer is yes," says Burnstein. "I think I need the separation to facilitate a pure focus on the task."

For surgeons, the ability to detach emotionally and focus on the task at hand is especially necessary when dealing with the fallout of surgical mistakes.

"Dealing with bad outcomes and errors is extremely difficult, especially in the early years of a surgical career, but not only then," says Burnstein. "There can be tremendous fallout (I would argue even PTSD in the worst cases) from making errors or even just the perception that you made an error. My personal behaviour has been sleeplessness, anxiety, reliving the decision-making moments, inner voices trying to calm me down with reminders that I am not perfect and that's okay, that I have to 'shake it off' and that I must learn from this.

"The shake-it-off manoeuvre, easier said than done, is the key to being successful at tomorrow's tasks. It gets a bit easier as you get older. It really helps if you have a few colleagues with whom you can talk and commiserate."

Burnstein, who teaches surgical residents, says surgeons are only just beginning to instruct formally how to deal with mistakes. Much more fundamental is how surgeons balance their focus and discipline for the operation with empathy for the patient.

"Now and then, I will find myself dealing with something much worse than was expected and the consequences for the patient and her family will certainly enter my mind, accompanied by the emotional response of sadness and anger," says Burnstein.

That's how Dr. Sid Schwab, a retired general surgeon and author and blogger felt the day he lost a teenage girl in the operating room. The teen had been in a sled being towed by her family car, which her parents were driving, when the car went around a corner.

"She got whiplashed into a concrete culvert," says Schwab.

"She passed out at the scene but they took her home and put her on the couch. Then she had a cardiac arrest. She had a pulse when they brought her in and you do everything you can for a little kid like that."

Schwab took the teenager to the operating room, but the accident had caused far too much damage. "It just fractured her liver so badly that there was not much we could do about it. To go out into the waiting room and tell the parents of a 15-year-old girl that you couldn't save her life and have them pounding on my chest and saying, 'What do you mean you couldn't save her?' That was pretty heavy."

Schwab recalls his eyes welling up with tears as he sutured up the dead girl. To surgeons, the operating room is a kind of safe haven from emotional attachment to the patient. It was there that Schwab could concentrate on trying to repair a teenage girl's mortally wounded liver without thinking about how her parents would feel when he had to tell them the surgery didn't save her.

But taking a patient to the operating room and subjecting her to the controlled violence that goes with incising, dissecting and cauterizing human tissue has to involve an emotional bond between surgeon and patient that begins in the surgeon's consulting room or at the bedside. The surgeon has to invest time in preparing for surgery, and invest emotionally in the patient.

Surgeons seldom talk about that bond. Still, they must feel it. And, they've invented a telling bit of medical slang that addresses perfectly the ambivalence they experience about feeling emotionally attached to their patients.

As I mentioned briefly at the beginning of the book, surgeons use the phrase peek-and-shriek, which describes taking a patient to the operating room, opening up the belly (peek), realizing the patient has a condition that cannot be fixed (shriek), and then closing the belly without fixing the problem.

"That is a very commonly used phrase," says Dr. Christian Jones, a fellow in surgical critical-care at Ohio State University Medical Center in Columbus. Jones learned it during his residency in general surgery at the University of Kansas Medical Center in Kansas City. "We write that down on our patient lists. All of us know what it means."

Jones says the worst example of peek-and-shriek he's ever seen happened with a patient he knew had cancer. "We opened the abdomen, and the entire small intestine was white. The walls of the intestines—every bit of them—were completely covered with tumour. We closed the abdomen. There was nothing we could do."

One of the most common peek-and-shrieks is of a woman with ovarian cancer. According to the American Cancer Society, ovarian cancer is the ninth most common cancer among women. This year alone, more than 22,000 American women will be diagnosed with ovarian cancer and more than 15,000 will die of it, making it much more deadly than breast, colon and prostate cancer.

The reason ovarian cancer is a common cause of peek-and-shrieks is that only about 20 percent are detected early enough to cure. The symptoms of ovarian cancer, which include bloating, pelvic or abdominal pain, trouble eating or feeling full quickly, and having to urinate frequently and urgently, are vague enough to be passed off by both patient and physician until it's too late for a cure. Or, there may be no symptoms at all.

"I think *peek-and-shriek* is a quick way of getting the message across that you encountered a disaster and found yourself to be useless," says Burnstein. "It's really damning of our skill set that we looked in and found nothing we could do. To make light of our uselessness, *peek-and-shriek* covers that."

Listening to Marcus Burnstein talk about it, I get the sense that if surgery means diving in with both feet, *peek-and-shriek* means dipping one's toe in the water of emotional investment. It's one thing for the surgeon to take on a critically ill patient knowing the odds of survival—much less recovery—are slim. It's quite another for the surgeon to take a carefully prepared patient to the OR not knowing what shocking discoveries lie ahead.

That's what happened to Dr. Raz Moola, now an OBGYN in Nelson, British Columbia, when he was a resident more than ten years ago. Moola was part of a team looking after a 20-something-year-old woman in her third trimester of pregnancy. The woman complained of abdominal pain, and had been to hospital several times.

Because of the risk of exposing the unborn child to radiation, a CT scan of the abdomen was out of the question. Several ultrasounds failed to show anything abnormal. Pain undiagnosed, the doctors decided the deliver the baby by Caesarean section and have a look inside the woman's belly.

"You open this woman's abdomen expecting that you are going to find a uterus and a baby," Moola recalls. "What we found were tumour deposits *everywhere*. It was clear that she had metastatic gastric cancer. Right then and there, you know what this woman's future is, you know what this child's future is—that the child is not going to have a mom. We were in total shock. It was a 'dear God' moment."

Christian Jones has had similar experiences. He and his colleagues once admitted an elderly man who was vomiting blood. The man had heart and lung disease and was a risky candidate for surgery. Jones says the team devised an audacious plan in which the stomach would be removed, and the esophagus and intestines would be left unattached for several weeks to give the old man's body a chance to heal. Meanwhile, he would be fed by IV drip.

"I was excited because I thought we could really help this guy," says Jones. "But as soon as we got him to the operating room and opened his belly, we saw that his entire small intestine had died. It was black and purple. We were shocked."

All Jones and his colleagues could do was close up the abdomen and keep the man as comfortable as possible. He died soon after.

"I was fully expecting that we were going to fix this guy," says Jones. "[Instead] we gave the family the worst news possible—not only could we not fix him, but nobody could fix him. I didn't use the term *peek-and-shriek* in that case. I don't know if that's because I did have that emotional attachment."

The therapeutic relationship between patient and surgeon—though shrouded in the mystique of operative procedures and sterile drapes—is as rich and as complex as that between any doctor and patient. Clearly, there are times when surgeons are more concerned than detached—just like the rest of us.

CHAPTER FOURTEEN

Circling the Drain

A heart attack is triggered by a sudden and complete blockage of a coronary artery. Starved of oxygen, the heart muscle convulses into a spasm of chaotic electrical activity called ventricular fibrillation, which causes the heart to stop beating. Without a timely electric shock from a defibrillator, irreversible brain damage ensues six to ten minutes later, followed by death.

Medical textbooks portray death much like that: in the cold, sterile language of pathophysiology. That's what we learn in medical school about human demise. It's only when we arrive on the hospital wards and in the ER that we discover the other side of death—the emotional side, the one that rips apart the hearts of loved ones.

/////////

"Brian, do you mind coming over to the resuscitation room for a minute?" a nurse working in my hospital asked me. I told her I'd come over as soon as I finished with a couple of patients in the ambulatory care room where we see cuts and sprains.

It was nearly three in the morning and I was tired. I'd done my time taking care of patients in the resuscitation (resus) room. If there's one thing ER physicians hate, it's getting pulled back into a job, a patient or an assignment you thought you were over and done with for your shift.

But I already knew that it was going to be different this time.

Two hours before the nurse asked me to come back to resus, paramedics had brought in an impossibly young Asian man who had suffered cardiac arrest while working the night shift in a factory. He had been complaining of pain in his upper abdomen and lower chest for a day or two, but passed it off as indigestion. During a meal break, he called his mother to say he wasn't feeling well. Half an hour later, he collapsed.

The paramedics wheeled him into the first bay in the resuscitation room in full cardiac arrest. One was doing CPR, a second was manually ventilating the man using a bag-valve-mask device. A third medic gave us a report.

"Approximately 30-year-old man collapsed while on duty at work," the paramedic told us in a rat-a-tat staccato. "Found in full cardiac arrest. CPR started at scene. V-fib on the monitor, shocked times four, given Epi times three, plus Vasopressin. Went into asystole and has been that way for twenty minutes."

Asystole meant the heart was showing no electrical activity. A flat line for twenty minutes—added to the time that he was in ventricular fibrillation—meant the man was essentially unsalvageable. Those were the cold, hard facts. But he looked far too young for this to be happening to him. You never want to stop trying to save a patient like that.

"I don't think there's any point in continuing," said my colleague. "I'm calling it."

Calling it is slang for stopping resuscitation efforts and pronouncing the patient dead.

Just like that, it was over.

I went back to the ambulatory care area of the ER where a growing horde of minor problems awaited me. But I kept thinking about the man who had just died, and how his family would react to hearing the news.

About an hour later, I glanced up from the desk to see a short Asian woman in her mid-fifties walk past. She was accompanied by two police officers. I knew right away that she was the dead man's mother.

I decided to follow them as they made a sharp right turn and headed down a long hallway, past the main nursing station, until they reached the fourth bay in the resus—the only bay with its own sliding door. Built to prevent infected patients from spreading germs, it also allows a private space for family members to see their dead loved one and to grieve.

As the woman and the two police officers approached the entranceway to resus 4, I spotted my colleague who had called the death. Breaking bad news is the most difficult thing we do in the ER. I asked my colleague if he wanted me there when he talked to the mother. As I expected, he brushed me off. There's a code among doctors in the ER: if it's your patient, it's your duty to tell the next of kin.

I backed away as my colleague introduced himself to the woman and escorted her into a room at the far end of the resuscitation stretchers. I lingered for a second as the woman disappeared into the room. The instant the door to the room slid shut, the screams began.

Loud, grief-stricken, hysterical screams filled the ER.

By the time the nurse asked me to look in on the woman, an hour had passed since my colleague had broken the news that her son was dead.

I approached the door to the resuscitation room, where the nurse was waiting for me. "We were hoping you could talk to her," she said.

"We've tried comforting her. She won't leave the bedside. It's like we can't reach her. We don't know what to do."

The room was dark as I walked in. The dead man was lying face up on the gurney, his eyes wide open. To the left of him stood his mother, flanked by two nurses who were holding her and trying in vain to soothe her. The woman was shaking her son's lifeless body and shouting at him to wake up, as if he were asleep.

That the woman could not get past this moment and face the future was totally understandable. I kept what I hoped was a stoic yet kind look on my face as I made my way slowly towards her.

Truth is, I was stalling. I had no idea what—if anything—I could do to help her.

///////

This was almost certainly the woman's first time seeing death up close. As a thirty-year veteran of the ER, I have seen it many times. Some patients—like the Asian man—arrive in full cardiac arrest the first time I set eyes upon them. Others die on my watch.

Despite my long experience, I always feel as if I'm rather inept at helping families deal with all things death. I'm not alone. As a profession, we find it difficult to talk to patients near the end of life about taking a pass on heroic measures. Telling next of kin about an unexpected death is the most difficult experience because you have to stay there and absorb that raw moment when they're processing the reality of what has happened. There is no training in med school or residency that prepares you for that.

If that's how I feel after thirty years on the job, imagine how residents and medical students feel. We'd never allow senior medical students or first-year residents to give it their best shot taking out your gall bladder without an experienced colleague there to provide support, if not take over. But when it comes to pronouncing someone dead in hospital, it's often the youngest and most inexperienced person on the team that gets the job.

Dr. Peter Kussin—the expert in medical slang at Duke University Hospital—also happens to be an authority on how to talk to patients who hover between life and death in the ICU, as well as to their families. He is trying to teach residents to follow in his footsteps—sometimes in vain.

"Have you listened to young physicians talk about end-of-life issues?" Kussin asks rhetorically. "I will sit there and let my residents sometimes lead the conversation. I want to bury my head in my hands, which I won't do, because that would be disrespectful to my young colleagues.

"They are devoid of the sort of communication skills that you need to do it. I tell them you've got to come and listen to old doctors with grey hair who've done this for twenty-five years like I did. And learn how they do it and model yourselves after them."

A young resident who could learn a thing or two from Dr. Kussin told me an illustrative story. He was once on call at a hospital when he was awakened at 4:30 a.m. to pronounce a patient dead. The 92-year-old man had been transferred to the hospital from a nursing home with symptoms of heart failure. It was his third hospital admission that year, and doctors suspected that he'd had a heart attack prior to being admitted this time.

The resident had never treated the man or met his family. As the resident on call, it was his job to pronounce the man dead. The hitch is that the young resident had never done it before.

"I called the senior resident and she said to listen to the heart and lungs for a minute," says the resident. "Look in their eyes to make sure their pupils are fixed and dilated. Test the pain reflex to make sure there is no response. And then fill out the death certificate."

It sounds as if the senior resident was schooling the newbie on how to put on a sling or an ankle wrap. From his account, she said nothing to him about how to inform the family, much less how to provide them with emotional support.

"I was kind of half asleep and I walked into the room," recalls the resident. "Two family members were crying. In my exhausted state, I asked them to leave the room, and I was left there with this man who had just died."

The resident says the patient was obviously dead. As he went through the motions of listening to the man's heart, another thought formed in his tired head. "The longer I listened, the longer I didn't have to go face the family behind the curtains," he confesses.

There are several aspects to this sorry situation that left the recent medical school graduate feeling embarrassed. One is that even though the patient was obviously near death when he was admitted, the hospital had stringent visiting hour procedures in effect. Only one visitor at a time was permitted in the patient's room. "It was so awful because the family wanted to be there when he died and they were kind of in an argument with the nursing staff," says the resident. "It was not a good way to die."

The other thing that bothered him was a near total disconnect between the mood of the family and that of the nurses. The resident discovered that when he looked for a quiet place to fill out the death certificate.

"I go to the nursing station and everyone's laughing," he says. The nurses weren't laughing about the death but they were having a good time. What's so bizarre about medicine is how you walk from the worst part in people's lives and then you enter the nursing station and I was laughing and joking with the nurses. I was cognizant of the fact that maybe the family can see me smiling now."

What the resident witnessed was the absence of any emotional identification between those at the nursing station who were laughing and the bereaved family. As I have argued, in the modern, post-Oslerian world of medicine, emotional detachment by health-care workers should be balanced by displays of genuine empathy. But to accomplish that, you have to care about your patients and their families in the first place.

I have no doubt that first experience pronouncing a patient dead will stick with the resident for the rest of his career.

"I'll probably never forget the looks on their faces and how I felt in that moment," he says. "I don't think I was afraid of the death or seeing the body. I was disappointed in myself that I wasn't present enough to give to the family at that time."

///////

Sooner or later, doctors have to get comfortable—or at least appear comfortable—with patients who die. That is an almost impossible task when the death is unexpected, as was the case with the Asian man. These are the deaths that generate shock from loved ones—a shock from which it is almost impossible to maintain an emotional distance.

In all such instances, medical slang helps doctors, nurses, paramedics and others who witness death up close maintain an emotional buffer. What's striking is just how often the slang is intended to be droll and ironic. *Discharged to God* and *discharged to heaven*—two commonly used bits of argot—come to mind. In hospital culture, there are only two possible outcomes for living patients: discharge to their own homes or transfer to another hospital or a nursing home. In fact, these are the only two outcomes anticipated for all patients admitted. Call doctors superstitious, but to talk about an anticipated death is to almost wish it. Thus, the phrase *discharged to heaven* suggests in an ironic way that the death was somehow planned and accomplished in much the same way that an appendix is removed.

A similar bit of slang refers to the death of a patient as *following up with pathology as an outpatient*. Once again, follow-up is a standard hospital transaction for all patients discharged—except of course for dead ones.

We prefer death to be expected and—more important—accepted by the family. That means family members cry a bit but are otherwise stoical about the loved one's demise. We hate screaming because bystanders may hear it and think we were negligent in the patient's care or, at the very least, negligent in our handling of the patient's family. When families accept death stoically, it means they move quickly from grief to taking care of operational details such as calling a funeral home. That enables us to move quickly to the next patient. Sounds cold, but it's true.

When a patient dies with no grieving relatives to deal with, so much the better. That's how it was with the first death I witnessed. It was 1979 and I was on my first rotation in internal medicine as a fourth-year medical student. I was assigned to a ward reserved for patients with gastrointestinal (GI) diseases such as peptic ulcer, hepatitis and the inflammatory bowel diseases Crohn's and ulcerative colitis.

Like many GI wards, this one was filled with patients in the final stages of alcoholic liver disease. One patient was a man in his early fifties whom I'll call Gustavo. After decades of drinking, he looked at least 70 and his liver tissue had been replaced with scar tissue. He had cirrhosis and now his liver was failing.

Gustavo had been admitted to the ward a day or two before I arrived for my first day on my internal medicine rotation. A textbook case, he had physical findings of cirrhosis galore. Gustavo was jaundiced to the point that his skin was bronzed. His huge belly was round and full of a watery liquid called ascites. If Dr. Peter Kussin had been looking after Gustavo, he'd have called him a Yellow Submarine.

Gustavo had a late-stage complication of cirrhosis called hepatic encephalopathy. Toxins that his liver was no longer able to eliminate were building up in his bloodstream. The toxins made Gustavo sleepy and often comatose.

Cirrhosis is irreversible. Even today the only remedy is a liver transplant. The first liver transplant had been performed in Denver, Colorado, back in 1963, but this option wasn't possible for Gustavo. They wouldn't become commonplace until the 1980s, when the surgical technique was perfected and the use of anti-rejection drugs such as cyclosporine became routine.

From my vantage point as a senior medical student, it didn't appear as if we were winning the battle to pull Gustavo back from the brink. Along with a junior resident, my senior and I would make rounds at eight in the morning. We would push a rolling chart rack along the hallway, stopping at each patient room long enough for a quick check. When we stopped at Gustavo's room, the ritual went like this:

"Good morning, Gustavo," the senior resident would say with a trace of irony as the team walked in.

"*Mmmrrrrr*," Gustavo would growl back, half awake.

"We're going to have a good day, Gustavo, aren't we?" my resident would reply in a tone of voice that sounded both ironic and condescending.

And with that, we would leave Gustavo's room and head off to see the next patient.

That ritual went on day after day without change. One morning near the end of my one-month rotation, my senior resident and I arrived in the morning only to find that Gustavo had suffered a fatal heart attack. The cardiac arrest team was packing up to leave as we arrived.

We stared at Gustavo's lifeless body. Quietly, the senior resident scolded Gustavo's lifeless form for drinking himself to death.

And with that, my senior resident walked out of Gustavo's room without a backward glance.

That was my first death: seemingly cold, lonely and cruel.

///////

Residents invent many slang terms to talk about the impending demise of patients. *Entering the drain* is slang for a hospitalized patient who is quite ill and could survive but is teetering on the brink of death. *Circling the drain* means the patient has entered the inevitable phase and can't be saved. *Crashing* means he's taken a sudden turn for the worse. *Crumping* is a synonym for crashing. *Fixing to die* is a term that implies that the patient has chosen his or her fate deliberately.

You get the picture. There are many such terms. They serve several purposes. One of the most important is to give a heads-up to the resident on call to expect that a lot of time and attention will be needed to save the patient's life and (if push comes to shove) to deal with grieving family.

Dr. Clarissa Burke, who did a residency in family medicine at McMaster University in Hamilton, Ontario, told me that phrases such as *circling the drain* imply that death is inevitable: "I don't know if that's a way of trying to remove our own responsibility from the situation or maybe even make us feel better about what's happening."

Such phrases usually get passed down from senior resident to junior and from junior to med student. Sometimes, they come from an attending physician. Dr. Rick Mann, who practises family medicine, told me a memorable example. "The one that has always stuck with me, unfortunately, is a staff physician who colloquially used to say about patients: 'Tell them not to buy any green bananas'—in the sense that they weren't going to be around to see them go ripe," said Mann.

As a resident in internal medicine in New York City back in the 1980s, respirologist Peter Kussin remembers sharing medical slang freely with his resident colleagues. Back then, two of Kussin's favourite slang terms for patients who were dying were PBAB, for "pine box at bedside," and the even more serious PBABLO, for "pine box at bedside, lid open."

"We would use those in our notes and our sign-outs," Kussin recalls. "So we'd say, Mr. Smith, Room 8322, PBAB, NTD—for "pine box at bedside, nothing to do." You have an intern who's got forty patients to cover. He knows that Mr. Smith doesn't need anything except end-of-life care."

But that was in New York City in the 1980s. Kussin wanted to find out whether the residents he teaches today at Duke use slang to talk about patients at the end of life.

Kussin says he once told a resident in the ICU "'I need you to meet with this family today. I'll meet with them tomorrow but I need you to hang crepe.' None of [the residents] had heard it. And that's a mild piece of medical slang."

Kussin was using the expression *hang crepe* to get the resident to prepare a patient's family for their loved one's impending death. He was also trying to make a connection with the resident—to let the resident know Kussin was there to share the emotional burden of telling the family.

One young physician remembers being on duty in the ER and seeing a 20-year-old man with osteosarcoma, an aggressive form of bone cancer that usually strikes teenagers. Only two-thirds of patients survive long-term. He recalls that the young man was receiving powerful chemotherapy drugs that lowered his white blood cell count and rendered his immune system vulnerable to attack by bacterial infection. The patient had a fever, an ominous sign that an infection had invaded his bloodstream.

"When I opened the door, it kind of hit [me] in the face," says the resident. "This patient looked very sick to me."

He started antibiotics and fluids by intravenous drip and transfused the young man with blood because the chemotherapy had also caused his hemoglobin to fall drastically. He referred the patient to the internal medicine team to be admitted. Medically, he did everything right. But he knew the young man was likely to die.

"You're sitting there with family members of a 20-year-old," says the resident. "They want you to tell them that everything is going be okay. And you want to tell them everything is going be okay. Instead, you have to find a middle ground and say things like you're going to do everything you can to make him feel better while trying not to lie to them."

Sometimes, we do what the resident did to be kind to the family. And sometimes, we do it to be kind to ourselves.

/////////

Dealing with death and its aftermath is one of the great emotional burdens that doctors take on when they enter the profession. You might think we would do almost anything to stave off death. Instead, more and more doctors take a tangible step to try to hasten death's arrival by securing from patients and loved ones permission to do nothing if and when death approaches and the heart stops. Doctors call that Do Not Resuscitate, or DNR.

In 1960, William Kouwenhoven, James Jude and Guy Knickerbocker of The Johns Hopkins University School of Medicine in Baltimore published an article in the *Journal of the American Medical Association* titled "Closed-Chest Cardiac Massage." It was the first to report on what would eventually become known as cardio-pulmonary resuscitation, or CPR.

The technique took off from there. The American Heart Association developed standards for health professionals on how to do CPR. By 1973, experts even recommended that the public be trained. The hope was that the widespread teaching of CPR to lay-people and the teaching of both CPR and more advanced techniques to health-care professionals could significantly reduce the 1,000 deaths from cardiac arrest that were then estimated to occur in the United States each day.

So far, that has not been the case. Most of the time, CPR doesn't work.

A 1983 paper in the *New England Journal of Medicine* reported that only thirty of 294 patients resuscitated at a teaching hospital were alive and well six months later. In a 2001 study published in the journal *Resuscitation*, Dr. Kamal Khalafi and co-authors wrote, "Instituting or continuing CPR in a great majority of these patients is futile. Families should be so advised."

From the earliest days, doctors fretted about doing CPR when it's futile. The American Heart Association published this warning in its standards for cardiopulmonary resuscitation and emergency cardiac care (ECC) in the *Journal of the American Medical Association*, in 1974:

Cardiopulmonary resuscitation is not indicated in certain situations, such as in cases of terminal irreversible illness where death is not unexpected or where prolonged cardiac arrest dictates the futility of resuscitation efforts. Resuscitation in these circumstances may represent a positive violation of an individual's right to die with dignity.

They didn't call it DNR back then. A 1976 article in the *New England Journal of Medicine* called it "orders not to resuscitate" (ONTR). Many hospitals use the slang term *Code Blue* to summon the cardiac arrest team to resuscitate a patient, so some doctors refer to an order not to resuscitate by the slang term *No Code*—for "no Code Blue." Some countries use the acronym DNI to signify "do not intubate," meaning the patient is not to receive a breathing tube or be placed on a ventilator. Other countries use the acronym NFR, for "not for resuscitation."

In 2005, the American Heart Association adopted the term DNAR, which stands for "do not attempt resuscitation," to reduce the unspoken implication that successful resuscitation is likely. More recently, some hospitals have called it AND, for "allow natural death." The term emphasizes that death is a natural consequence of a disease or injury.

Call it DNR or No Code or whatever euphemism you happen to like. It's a transaction between doctor and patient that is like no other in all of medicine. In almost every other aspect, you see a doctor who proposes a treatment and invites you to consent to it or refuse it. You don't get to demand it. Worried about breast cancer because you've seen too many friends fall victim to the disease? Try ordering your surgeon to perform a double mastectomy. You're more than likely to be sent to a psychiatrist than get the surgery. Try forcing a heart specialist do an angioplasty. That won't happen either. Only the doctor decides if the treatment you want is appropriate.

The only exception is resuscitation, including CPR. Shocking the heart, ventilating and a whole host of other measures are the only treatments in the arsenal that doctors *have to* perform unless you give us permission not to.

How the heck did that happen? Blame it on the tragic story of Karen Ann Quinlan. In April 1975, Quinlan, a 21-year-old college student, became comatose after arriving home from a bar, where she had attended a friend's birthday celebration. It's believed the coma was caused by a combination of alcohol, the sedative diazepam and the painkiller dextropropoxyphene. Quinlan was admitted to Newton Memorial Hospital in New Jersey, where she was placed on a ventilator. Eventually, her doctors diagnosed her as being in a persistent vegetative state.

What makes Quinlan's case a seminal one is that her parents asked the hospital to take their daughter off the ventilator and allow her to die. The hospital turned down the parents' request, setting the stage for a battle in the courts that attracted attention worldwide. In the end, the New Jersey Supreme Court sided with the parents. In 1976, Quinlan was taken off the ventilator. She lived for another nine years off life support, until she succumbed to pneumonia in 1985.

The 1976 *New England Journal of Medicine* article cited the Quinlan case as a precedent that the wishes of patients and family members must be paramount. From that point on, full resuscitation became the default option in the absence of clear directives to the contrary.

Until that point, resuscitation was largely the prerogative of physicians and hospitals. The Quinlan case turned it into a mutual decision. Paradoxically, it was Quinlan's parents who wanted to turn off the ventilator that was keeping their daughter alive against the objections of her doctors. Today, family members are commonly insisting on CPR as doctors fight against it.

There are several reasons doctors would rather chew glass than do CPR on most patients. For the vast majority of hospitalized patients, resuscitation is futile. Your loved one is admitted to hospital with metastatic lung cancer. Death is inevitable and probably imminent. But if your loved one's heart stops, and you haven't signed a DNR, I have no choice but to do CPR and put him or her on a ventilator.

That's the obvious reason. The less obvious ones are buried within the culture of medicine. Doctors hate being ordered to render any treatment; if the patient or family are giving the orders, so much the worse.

Most doctors I know would love to be able to decide on their own whether you or a loved one should get resuscitated. In the current system, that's not possible. So we go for the next best thing: *getting the DNR*—that is, subtly persuading patients and families to not demand resuscitation efforts.

Today, hospitals have a DNR form that patients or their substitute decision-makers are asked to sign. From a distance, a DNR discussion looks like a negotiation. In reality, it's a dance in which we doctors hope to lead patients and their families to see the futility and agree with the doctors.

"Several of us have referred to it as 'closing the deal,'" says Peter Kussin. "If patients heard us or their families heard us describe it that way, they would not like it. I would not blame them for not liking it. It reflects that the level of communication that occurs in ICUs and in people with advanced illness is usually pressured by time. Physicians are uncomfortable with it."

And who do we dispatch to get the DNR? In a teaching hospital, we send in rookies. As is the case with pronouncing the patient deceased, it's often the most junior member of the medical team who has the task of getting the DNR from a patient newly diagnosed with a life-threatening condition (or the next of kin). Often, the discussion takes place in a cubicle or a hallway in the ER.

A senior medical student remembers doing an admission history and a physical on an 81-year-old man who had come to hospital complaining of loss of appetite and a weight loss of twenty pounds. A chest X-ray showed the man had a large collection of fluid inside his chest cavity between the inside of the chest wall and a lung. Given the man's loss of appetite and weight, the most likely and most ominous cause was cancer.

In the Bunker, the student's senior resident gave him his marching orders. "This was a medically futile situation," the student recalls. "The resident just kind of handed me these two sheets and said, 'Go get the DNR,' like a rite of passage."

At some hospitals, a DNR form is a single sheet that asks whether the patient wants CPR or to be put on a ventilator should the need arise. More and more, hospitals like the one where the student was on duty that night have a multi-page DNR form with so many options it reminds me of beverage choices at Starbucks.

The student went to visit the man, who was alone. The senior resident had told him to get a DNR, but there was an important detail the student had to take care of first. He had to tell the man it was highly likely that he had cancer and that he probably did not have long to live.

"You can imagine that this person had just been broken the news that he has cancer," says the student. "Then you're asking him what he wants to do if his heart stops. I don't think people are in the right mindset by any means to make that decision at that time."

Did the man want a breathing tube? Check. An IV? Check. Blood work? Check. Antibiotics in case of an infection? Check, check and check. The more options the student discussed, the more bewildered the patient became.

"We kind of fumbled through it," says the student, cringing at the memory. "I was left with the feeling that this was inappropriate to do under these circumstances. This was not offering him an option of dignified care."

In fairness, the doctor-to-be had to conduct a conversation of that import while answering pages and rushing off to do other referrals. Still, conscience or not, he had a job to do.

"The resident really had this expectation that I was going to come back with the DNR because it was outrageous for this person with metastatic cancer to receive resuscitative measures," says the student.

In the end, he says he got the DNR, and a high five from the senior resident when he returned to the Bunker with the signed form—and with a lot of personal misgivings. "I really hate the menu option of 'How do you want to die?'" he says.

These days, getting the DNR is more about filling out paperwork than having a heartfelt conversation like the one the student wished he had had with his patient.

Few have thought more about what that particular student as well as multitudes of students and residents have struggled with than Dr. Peter Kussin. "I've certainly said it myself: 'Did you get the DNR order?' or something like that," says Kussin. "It jangles a little bit because it's a little stark reminder of how we've de-emotionalized or depersonalized the situation."

In hospital corridors, there are lots of misgivings about the way we deal with DNRs.

In a trenchant commentary published in 2011 in the *Journal of General Internal Medicine*, Dr. Jacqueline Yuen and colleagues wrote that DNR discussions occur too infrequently and often are delayed until it is too late for patients to participate in the decision-making. They also made the troubling observation that the more a hospital serves up high-tech, cutting-edge treatments, the less inclined it is to sit down with patients and discuss their end-of-life wishes. More disturbing is the authors' observation that for-profit hospitals that serve up the most costly treatments also have lower rates of DNR.

To me, this sounds like a cash cow being milked to death.

The authors blamed doctors and hospital policies—even the

Joint Commission, the organization that accredits more than 20,000 health-care organization and programs in the United States—for not informing patients and families of the options for resuscitation available to them. They also called out medical schools and residency programs for not requiring that students and doctors-in-training receive formal training on how to talk to families about DNR.

I know all about that. Ten years ago, I treated a man with severe Parkinson's disease. He could no longer speak for himself, but he had a devoted sister who spoke eloquently on his behalf. He was close to the end of his life, and the sister wanted him to be admitted to hospital and treated with dignity. Instead of seeing the loving sibling that she was, I saw her as just another demanding relative who was asking for more from me than I had time to deliver.

I acceded to her request and referred her brother to be admitted to the internal medicine team. But I was cold and insensitive to her. After the patient died some time later, the sister met with me and took me to task for my attitude. We came to an understanding, but the memory still stings because I failed to support her emotionally.

Yuen and her co-authors called for better guidelines on DNR from the Joint Commission and better training for students, residents and attending physicians. They also liked an idea that was part of original health reform legislation proposed by President Barack Obama during his first term in office—to pay doctors a bonus for handling DNR discussions well. Unfortunately, the notion of providing payment to doctors for conversations with patients and families about end-of-life care led critics of the health-care reform bill to accuse the government of hatching a scheme to limit health care to seniors by setting up what critics referred to as "death panels."

I think end-of-life discussions should happen at a time when patients can ponder their wishes without feeling pressure to sign a form. Advance directives, sometimes called advance health-care directives or living wills, are written instructions about what people want done regarding their health if illness or incapacity make them unable to decide for themselves.

So far, few patients want them. A 2012 study found fewer than one in five elderly patients who visited the ER had advance directives.

All of which means DNR discussions in hospitals under highly stressful circumstances will be the norm for some time to come. Just starting his career, Dr. Nathan Stall is already disillusioned that end-of-life conversations have been reduced to getting the DNR. "I actually hate it now and this is someone who believes that this is such an important thing to do," says the aspiring geriatrician. "I think the pendulum has swung so far to the other side that it's just the most awkward conversation."

Doctors have long had a sneaky way of avoiding altogether those awkward conversations about DNR: Let the family think the doctors are doing a full cardiac arrest procedure when they have no intention of doing so.

The slang term is *Slow Code*. It means pretending to try and pull the patient back from the brink. In a real Code Blue, you drop everything and run to the patient's bedside. In a Slow Code, you walk, stroll or saunter. You're slow to arrive on the scene, slow to check for signs of unresponsiveness, slow to check for a pulse and slow to do every intervention, from CPR to defibrillation. It's a play for time until it's acceptable to pronounce the patient dead.

Slow Code is also known by the slang terms *Show Code, Hollywood Code* and *Light Blue*. I've also heard it referred to as *Blue Light*, named after a popular beer brewed by the Labatt Brewing

Company Ltd. Blue Light is a nice pun; like the beer, a Slow Code is a pale, low-calorie version of the real thing.

The first person to introduce me to Slow Code was a senior resident in internal medicine. One day, he announced to us that if and when a certain patient's heart stopped, the code would be a slow one. The day the man arrested, the cardiac arrest team arrived to find the senior resident by the bedside, taking the man's pulse in a very leisurely way. I remember that he announced to the residents who had arrived breathlessly that they could pack up and leave. They didn't object.

On that occasion, the senior resident called it a Slow Code out loud. However, in my experience, most clinicians who use the tactic don't name it; they just do it. It's very easy to telegraph that a Slow Code is in play by rolling one's eyes or by speaking the patois of cardiac resuscitation in a tone of voice that conveys an ironic meaning.

There are almost no statistics on the frequency of Slow Codes. However, in a 2012 article published in the journal *Virtual Mentor*, Dr. Edwin Forman, a pediatric hematologist and oncologist, and Rosalind Ladd, a visiting scholar in philosophy at Brown University in Providence, Rhode Island, wrote that "many medical students, residents, and other medical staff learn the elements of a *slow code* early in their clinical years."

The thing about a Slow Code is that it can't happen without the tacit agreement of every professional involved. The objections of even one of the doctors or nurses involved would raise the serious spectre of a complaint to hospital authorities, regulators, perhaps even the police. The absence of frequent whistleblowers tells me that a lot of people on the front lines think a Slow Code is the right thing to do—even if thought leaders disagree.

In 1992, Jessica Muller, a professor of medicine at the University of California at San Francisco, wrote an article in *Social Science &*

Medicine in which she referred to Slow Codes as "deplorable, dishonest and inconsistent with established medical principles."

The sixth edition of the *American College of Physicians Ethics Manual,* published in 2012, says this: "Because they are deceptive, half-hearted resuscitation efforts ('slow codes') should not be performed." The fifth edition of the authoritative textbook *Clinical Ethics* calls Slow Codes "dishonest, crass dissimulation, and unethical." In a 2010 article in the journal *Pediatrics,* Eric Kodish of the department of bioethics at the Cleveland Clinic condemned the practice of Slow Codes by saying that "charades are not acceptable when it comes to life-and-death matters."

Not everyone agrees. In a 2011 article published in the *American Journal of Bioethics,* Dr. John Lantos, a pediatrician and bioethicist, and Dr. William Meadow, a neonatologist and bioethicist, wrote that the "misunderstood and unfairly denigrated" Slow Code "may be appropriate and ethically defensible in certain clinical situations."

For instance, suppose family members understand that death is imminent and inevitable, but just can't sign a DNR form because to them it feels like playing God? In that scenario, Lantos and Meadow recommend that doctors *not* seek the family's explicit consent for a DNR. Instead, they recommend leaving the conversation deliberately vague and ambiguous so as to relieve the family of the burden of making a difficult decision and leave the doctors the option to act *as if* a DNR had been signed.

In a 2011 article published in the *Ochsner Journal,* Dr. Joseph Breault talks about his experiences during the early days of the HIV epidemic, when patients usually died of opportunistic infections. He wrote that his patients—who knew their fate because they'd seen it happen to many of their contemporaries—were quite comfortable with DNRs. Their family members were a different story. "Sometimes families thought they were being asked to render a death sentence," Breault recalls. Breault concluded that when it comes to death, language matters. Today, he prefers the term *allow natural death*, or AND.

What rankles with critics of Slow Codes the most is that the practice deceives patients and their families. So what? Lantos and Meadow might argue. In their article, they wrote that deception regarding CPR is "the tip of a vast iceberg of deceptiveness that pervades ICUs. . . .In the ICU, patients and their families are rarely told about or offered every possible intervention that could be used to prolong the life of a loved one. Nor are they explicitly asked to explicitly authorize the withholding of those interventions."

Lantos and Meadow are absolutely right. Even when a Full Code resuscitation is supposed to be done, patients and families aren't asked how long the code should go on before pronouncing the patient dead, what drugs to use and how many times the heart should be shocked, if at all.

While doctors believe CPR is usually futile, many families insist on it nonetheless. Lantos and Meadow blame the fact that Code Blue has been made famous as a dramatic device in television and film— and a highly inaccurate one at that.

In 1996, a trio of doctors briefly turned the *New England Journal of Medicine* into a magazine for TV critics with a review of CPR as portrayed on shows such as *ER, Chicago Hope* and *Rescue 911.* The authors found that three-quarters of the TV patients were shocked back to life, and two-thirds apparently lived long enough to be discharged from hospital—figures far removed from any concept of reality. If my heart stops, let it stop on the set of a TV show!

Lantos and Meadow postulate that TV and movie portrayals of CPR have reinforced the value of CPR—either as a way to save life or as a symbolic expression of the commitment not to give up on the patient. Thus, the authors recommend placating families by carrying out a "short, symbolic trial of CPR."

The word *trial* makes it sound like a clinical experiment. What Lantos and Meadow are talking about isn't CPR as treatment but as theatre. If the doctor thinks it's futile, then doing it so as not to appear to give up is—in my opinion—an act of physical cruelty on the patient.

What's even more bizarre about this suggestion is that it has some very respected proponents. In 2013, Dr. Robert Truog, a pediatric ICU doctor at Boston Children's Hospital, wrote a provocative article in the *New England Journal of Medicine* in which he defended the use of full-bore resuscitative measures on a two-year-old child with a devastatingly fatal degenerative disease. Though utterly futile, when the child's heart stopped he received a Full Code resuscitation, complete with CPR. Truog wrote that the resuscitation made one nurse battle the urge to throw up.

What's astonishing is that Truog wrote that he did it not for the child *but for his parents,* who viewed a Full Code as a valiant struggle to live against impossible odds. The intensivist wrote that when the child's father saw bruises and puncture wounds—the detritus of multiple failed attempts to establish a central venous line—he said: "I want to thank you. I can see from this that you really tried; you didn't just give up and let him die."

If I were the father, I might instead have thought about calling in the police to press charges of assault and battery on a defenceless child. But clearly my mindset is different from that of the father depicted in Truog's account.

I think we should invent a new slang term for what Lantos and Meadow proposed and what Truog actually did. Let's call it *CPR theatre* after another slang term, *hand-washing theatre*, a recent bit of argot that refers to a doctor entering a patient's hospital room and holding up hands glistening with the residue of alcohol rub. The purpose of hand-washing theatre is to show skeptical patients and their families that one's hands are free of germs.

Truog argued that the needs of the parents are "clinically and ethically significant," especially given the fact it is they who, as part of the grieving process, will bear the guilt for not having tried to save their child. That they might also feel guilt for subjecting their son to a futile attempt at resuscitation seems lost on the good doctor though obvious to me.

In an odd sort of way, the approach to CPR has become a case of medicine imitating art imitating medicine. At one point, recognizing a winning dramatic device, film and television writers and producers borrowed Code Blue from the world of medicine. They torqued the success rate of CPR for dramatic effect, and in so doing convinced the public that it was a lifesaver. That got the public to demand a mostly futile procedure, which in turn has forced medical practitioners to do it—or at least to look like they're doing it—futile or not.

//////

CPR theatre and the Hollywood Code symbolize the failure of doctors to communicate with patients and families. The obvious solution is better communication.

While visiting Duke University Hospital, I was told that Dr. Peter Kussin and a retired colleague were known affectionately as The Terminator and The Closer—not because they were aggressive about withdrawing life support but because they love helping families in their hour of greatest need. Both earned reputations for being able to get patients and their families to see the prognosis and the futility of aggressive, death-delaying treatments with the crystal clarity that comes with compassion and a strong command of accurate medical information.

Kussin honed his expertise in the ICU, where it's up to the doctors and nurses to talk to the patient's family—not about a DNR but about something a lot more touchy: stopping the things that are keeping the patient alive, such as ventilators and the intravenous drips that hold the powerful medications that maintain the patient's blood pressure. It's called "withdrawal of care."

Withdrawal of care is an increasingly important topic of conversation in the ICU, where a growing number of older patients with chronic heart failure and chronic obstructive lung disease get admitted for a last gasp at survival, both literally and figuratively. Often, families fail to grasp that their loved one is at or near the end of life, preferring to see a ventilator and intravenous drips as hopeful signs. And that's not the only factor that keeps families from grasping that the end is close.

"It's well documented that overwhelmed, stressed families or patients in the midst of a critical illness remember little and process less," says Kussin.

Talking is not enough; the challenge is to get patients and family members to understand the options well enough to make an informed choice. Kussin has thought a great deal about that. After all, you don't get to be called The Closer if you don't have a few decent pitches in your arsenal. "You have to be very careful, but humour definitely has a place," he says. "I use the term 'Hail Mary pass' all the time." *Hail Mary pass* is a slang term used in professional football to refer to a long forward pass thrown by a quarterback in the dying seconds of a football game—a desperation move to try to score a last-second touchdown that wins or at least ties the game.

"It's a metaphor that anyone with any level of understanding of popular culture or living in this century or the last one will understand," says Kussin. "It affords hope. It shows that I am doing something with some small degree of hope that it will be successful. But then, I'm also preparing the groundwork for the [likelihood] that ball is going to be intercepted or fall dead in the end zone."

I can't recall ever reading a single medical article or textbook that recommended using sports metaphors to obtain informed consent. I asked Kussin if such a metaphor might be taken the wrong way. "I don't think it's disrespectful to the severity of the illness," says Kussin. "I think people see me as being maybe a little more human than being an automaton decision-maker or expert."

If it works, then Kussin is much further ahead of the game than most health professionals I know. When we don't communicate well with patients and families, we leave them feeling alone and abandoned during the most difficult days of their lives.

Doctors and nurses feel that sense of emotional abandonment as well through a phenomenon called moral distress. Moral distress was first defined by the ethicist Dr. Andrew Jameton of the University of Nebraska Medical Center as "a phenomenon in which one knows the right action to take, but is constrained from taking it." The concept of moral distress was first described among nurses. A 2000 study published in the journal *Nursing Ethics* found that one in three nurses experience moral distress, particularly around end-of-life issues. A survey of 760 nurses published in 1993 in the *American Journal of Public Health* found that nearly half of those surveyed said they had acted against their conscience in providing care to patients who were terminally ill.

Moral distress can lead to burnout. A 1994 study published in the *Western Journal of Nursing Research* found that just under half of nurses said moral distress compelled them either to leave a nursing job or to leave the profession altogether. Most telling is the impact of moral distress on patient care. Numerous studies have shown that nurses who experience this form of psychological damage spend less time with patients.

Although much of the literature on moral distress focuses on nurses, it turns out that other health professionals are vulnerable. A

2009 study published in the *American Journal of Surgery* documented moral distress among third-year medical students. Ryan Herriott, himself a third-year medical student, chronicled the problem of moral distress among his classmates in a blog post on healthydebate.ca. Herriott said the factors contributing to students' moral distress included the need to be seen by residents and fellow medical students as a team player. When being a good member of the team requires that doctors give patients short shrift, we feel moral distress.

That's what the senior medical student was struggling with when his senior resident ordered him to "get the DNR" on an elderly man with end-stage cancer. The student wanted to help the man come to grips with dying; instead, he was consumed with getting the man to sign the paperwork.

Sometimes, moral distress comes from wanting to do the right thing but not having the time to do it. Often, though, it's not time that's the problem but lack of training. As health professionals, physicians are *expected* to be caring people by nature. Astonishing though you may find it, most doctors find it difficult to respond to their patients empathically. These days, empathy is not a treasured skill in medicine. A near-perfect grade-point average and a high score on the Medical College Admission Test (MCAT) are the ingredients of a successful application.

By the time you finish med school and residency, you have absorbed the unspoken message that as a physician you are judged to be either brilliant in a clinical sense or empathetic—but not both. With a choice like that, it's a wonder anyone would want to be seen as empathetic.

Like the senior medical student, I learned how to break bad news badly, and it ate away at me from the inside.

Then, one day, I had an epiphany from a master who taught me how to respond to patients with a dose of empathy. My teacher was my friend and sometime mentor, the late Dr. Robert Buckman. Buckman wrote many books aimed at helping people like me take better care of patients. His textbook *How to Break Bad News: A Guide for Health Care Professionals* is a standard text at many colleges and universities. Likewise, Buckman shared his wisdom with the lay public with books such as *CANCER is a Word, Not a Sentence*; *What You Really Need to Know About Cancer* and *I Don't Know What to Say: How to Help & Support Someone Who is Dying.*

Buckman was an expert without peer at communicating with patients—a skill that came from having a good heart and from an early brush with death. In 1979, Buckman was diagnosed with dermatomyositis, an autoimmune disease that causes inflammation of the skin, muscles and other parts of the body. His experience as a patient taught him how important it was to see the world from the patient's point of view, a lesson he put to excellent use when he recovered.

Buckman taught me that empathy is all about giving patients and family members the space and the approval to feel what they feel. He made me realize that doctors get into trouble breaking bad news because they pay too much attention to their own emotional distress to let the patient or family member talk about theirs.

The lesson has wide implications. As a profession, we spend far too much time talking *around* patients who are dying and not enough talking *with* patients who are dying.

Buckman said it's possible to teach physicians how to respond empathically to patients just as you show them how to set a broken bone or suture a cut—one patient and one family member at a time. "The black art to breaking bad news is very simple," Buckman told me on *White Coat, Black Art.* "And it's much more simple than you thought it was."

He said the first step to breaking bad news is not to blurt out the news but to listen to the patient or family to find out first what they already know. The second step is to deliver the bad news as sensitively as possible. The third step is to respond to every emotion the patient or loved one expresses. For example, if the doctor tells a patient that she has cancer and the patient refuses to believe it, Buckman said it's wrong to argue with her; the correct response is to acknowledge the patient's disbelief.

"You acknowledge the fact that it is difficult to for her to believe it," said Buckman. "The actual words that you use don't matter. The action of the empathic response is to acknowledge the emotion in what the other person says, and that's what you do."

///////

I stood close to the short Asian woman in her mid-fifties as she shook her dead son and cried out to him to wake up.

Buckman's words rang through my mind as I put a hand on the woman's shoulder. "Difficult to believe he's gone," I said.

She ignored me completely as she continued shaking her son. "Wake up!" she yelled at him in a language I could not understand. Her voice was getting hoarse.

"It must be so hard for you to believe that your son could die like this," I said.

Again, the mother didn't acknowledge what I said. I wasn't sure whether she knew I was in the room, much less speaking to her.

I must have tried a dozen different ways to acknowledge the woman's disbelief that her son was dead. I knew that I had failed to form an empathic bond with her. It was nearly four in the morning. I was tired to the bones and I needed to sleep. The two nurses who had spent an hour trying in vain to comfort the woman and to help her to move forward looked exhausted, both physically and emotionally.

Why wasn't I connecting with her?

Somewhere, in the midst of this horrific scene, it occurred to me that I had failed because all the while I had been responding not to the mother's distress but to mine. The nurses and I wanted the woman to acknowledge that her son was dead and to move on. We wanted that because that's what *we* needed. But that was not what she wanted.

Now, I could hear Buckman's voice urging me to acknowledge what the mother was doing. But what was the right thing to say?

"You keep shaking your son," I heard myself saying. The woman didn't react to my words. She kept on shaking him. What I said sounded weird, yet it felt right. In a simple way, I was acknowledging what she was doing.

"You keep shaking your son," I repeated, this time more confidently. "You think that if you shake him hard enough, you will wake him up. But you can't, because he's gone."

With that, the woman stopped shaking her son and stopped calling out to him.

For the first time since she had seen her son's lifeless body, the woman sat down in a chair and began to sob.

CHAPTER FIFTEEN

Slang Police

D octors have invented hundreds—perhaps thousands—of slang terms that portray patients and their attitudes, fears, hidden agendas and even their appearance in unflattering terms. Call it the nature of medical argot, but rarely if ever do doctors invent words that compliment the people they care for.

That the slang I uncovered exists in such volume and is spoken by so many doctors and other health professionals can mean only one thing. If you're old, demented, frail, mentally ill, overly anxious about your health, morbidly obese, addicted, in police custody or if you just call on us too often, we're not keen on having you as a patient.

And that is a growing problem for doctors. That's because the "undesirables" I just listed have rapidly become the typical inhabitants of hospitals. Older patients are but one example. The United States is adding 10,000 people to the ranks of seniors each and every day. Obese patients are another growing problem. A 2012 report by the Robert Wood Johnson Foundation says that by the year 2030 half of U.S. adults will be obese. Patients with substance abuse are also growing in number. In 2008, the National Institute on Drug Abuse estimated that 14 percent of all patients admitted to hospital have alcohol- or drug-abuse and addiction disorders, which accounts for nearly 20 percent of all Medicaid hospital costs.

Add them up, and in 2012, the CDC says, chronic diseases—the ones I listed, plus others—accounted for 75 percent of the $2.5 trillion spent each year on health care in the U.S.

Does that mean doctors have given up on patients? Hardly. It's just that we're highly selective. My colleagues still love to shock hearts back into normal rhythm, swap unhealthy lungs and livers with healthy ones, unclog blocked coronary arteries, not to mention cut, zap and drug cancers into remission. These are neat and tidy patients for whom we furnish happy endings. That we get to play the hero only adds to the glory. These are the patients we tell triumphant stories about.

Increasingly, though, patients like these are in the minority. Today's typical patient makes many of my colleagues flinch.

Why don't we like them? Different patients illustrate different aspects of the problem. Cockroaches—patients who come back again and again to the ER and other parts of the hospital—represent failure to doctors. After all, if we'd helped them the first time, why would they need to come back? Swallowers, likewise, represent the failure of the repeat customer—plus the added frustration that comes from being unable to know what makes them tick, much less help them.

We invent the slang terms *status dramaticus* for anxious patients because they test our ability to quell their anxiety and *C-section consent form* to vent our frustration with patients who want a say in how things go during labour and delivery.

We dislike bariatric or morbidly obese patients for complex reasons. Most health professionals receive little education to counteract society's overt prejudice against overweight people. Doctors are no better than the rest of society about seeing obesity as a condition that is entirely self-inflicted. And although bariatric-rated lifts, stretchers and other equipment for heavy patients are on the market, many hospitals fail to purchase them.

Likewise, we don't like GOMERs or FTDs for complex reasons. Dementia means they can't answer our questions thoughtfully, if at all. In a health-care system that prizes speed and productivity, old patients slow us down. Most doctors have little if any substantive training in how to recognize many of the unique health challenges facing frail older patients. I suspect we also dislike seniors because they're manifestations of a future few of us look forward to. And some of us wish they would just die because we believe their continued existence wastes precious health-care dollars and offends the notion of a dignified end to life.

The reasons we invent slang such as *cowboy* and *flea* that disparages colleagues are somewhat different. Insecurity over income and status are among the factors that motivate doctors lower down on the food chain to disparage colleagues who are seen as being higher up. A slang term such as *hypervaginosis* is used to reinforce cohesion within a group and isolation of outliers, as well as dominance by the group's leadership.

These musings are my opinions on the subject gleaned from more than twenty years as a keen observer of the culture of modern medicine. I doubt many of my colleagues would agree—at least publicly. Let me go one step further. I'd say the vast majority of doctors have given scarce thought to what I'm talking about. That slang exists in such abundance is proof that it's easier for front-line doctors to express frustration with patients and with each other than it is to talk about what makes them frustrated in the first place.

To be sure, lots of articles have been published in medical journals about what medicine calls the "difficult patient." Typically, it's someone who argues constantly with doctors about treatment choices or who never follows the doctor's advice. But those articles almost always focus on the patient as a difficult person. Almost never do they focus on doctors who dislike their patients.

One doctor who has written openly about dislike for patients is

Don Dizon, a cancer specialist and director of medical oncology at the Program in Women's Oncology at Women & Infants' Hospital of Rhode Island. In a March 2013 blog published in *ASCO Connection*, the professional networking site for the American Society of Clinical Oncologists, Dizon wrote at length about a woman in her forties with a newly diagnosed breast cancer who at her first meeting with Dizon got angry that the cancer doctor wasn't already up to speed on her clinical history.

In his blog post, Dizon says he tried to empathize with the woman. "It must be really shocking to be here," he told her. "No one our age expects something like this to happen."

The patient responded with more anger. "Just concentrate on the facts, please," she replied. "I don't need your pity. What I want is your expertise."

Dizon says the relationship went downhill from there. The doctor began to dread his patient's appointments. He sought the support of his colleagues. "I don't like this woman," he told his partners. But they weren't with him at all.

"You should not say that," one of them told Dizon. "It's not her fault she has cancer, and people cope in very different ways."

Despite the difficulties, Dizon didn't end the doctor-patient relationship, as often happens. Instead, he forged a more realistic relationship with his patient by acknowledging and processing his dislike.

"Medicine requires us to do what's in the best interest of our patients, to 'do no harm.' It does not compel us, however, to 'like' everyone we treat."

It's both brave and unusual of Dizon to admit he didn't like the woman. Far more common is the reaction of knee-jerk admonishment from the colleague who articulated to Dizon an unwritten rule in medicine: *You never hate your patients, because you are better than they are, and admitting those feelings says you aren't.* Maybe it's me,

but I sensed something more than disapproval from the colleague—
something closer to rejection, a sort of punishment for being honest.

There are strong parallels between the reaction of Dizon's colleague and the response of organized medicine to medical argot and
the pejorative attitudes the slang words represent.

/////////

Twenty years ago, a new force bubbled up in hospital and medical
school corridors that threatened to eradicate slang from the known
medical universe. It was an earnest movement with the Orwellian
name of "medical professionalism." According to an article published
in 2000 in the journal *Academic Medicine* by early acolyte Dr. Herbert
Swick, then the executive director of the Institute of Medicine and
Humanities, a joint program of the University of Montana and St.
Patrick Hospital and Health Sciences Center in Missoula, Montana,
"Medical professionalism consists of those behaviors by which we—
as physicians—demonstrate that we are worthy of the trust bestowed
upon us by our patients and the public, because we are working for
the patients' and the public's good."

Swick listed nine attributes of medical professionalism, including this one: "Physicians evince core humanistic values, including
honesty and integrity, caring and compassion, altruism and empathy,
respect for others, and trustworthiness."

Dr. Richard Cruess and his wife and professional partner, Dr.
Sylvia Cruess, have become internationally recognized leaders in
this burgeoning field. In 1995, both left stellar careers in academic
medicine to do research on professionalism. "What we try and do in
medical school and during residency training is inculcate the values
of the physician so they come to think, act and feel like doctors," says
Richard Cruess.

In sociological terms, what the Cruesses are talking about is helping medical students and residents forge what's known as a professional identity.

"So what they do is they play the role," says Richard Cruess. "They analyze what the role is supposed to be."

"And they analyze it by what they see around them in their role models," says Sylvia Cruess.

"This is not bright people consciously doing this," says Richard Cruess. "Most of the time, it's intuitive. You're in a culture where there are certain norms and you adhere to those norms."

And where does this professional identity come from? The Cruesses say some of it goes back to Hippocrates himself. The Hippocratic Oath is filled with ethical standards such as promising not to harm patients and keeping what the patient tells the doctor secret.

When I went to medical school in the 1970s, there were no courses on medical professionalism. It was the same for Richard and Sylvia Cruess, who trained before me. Even the word *professionalism* was seldom used. I wanted to find out why it became such a priority in the late 1980s and early '90s.

Richard Cruess says at the time there was a general feeling that several forces were threatening medicine's traditional concept of professionalism. Sylvia Cruess says one factor was the explosion in medical technology. "We had many more technical things in our armamentarium," she says. "The more technical you become, the less you remember that it's a human being you're working with."

Richard Cruess says another factor that underscored the need to spell out the principles of medical professionalism was the growing heterogeneity of doctors. "Life was much simpler in those days," he says. "You have to remember that most of our society was much more homogeneous. The values were Judeo-Christian. Those values corresponded much more to the values of the professional. There were very few minorities in medical school. Our professors were more homogeneous."

Since everyone came from pretty much the same religious and cultural background—and shared the same values—it was assumed that everyone adhered to the same notions of professionalism. That's certainly not true anymore.

Another factor is economic. In Swick's article in *Academic Medicine*, he wrote that medical professionalism is "a way to respond to the corporate transformation of the U.S. health-care system."

The corporate transformation of medicine in the 1970s and '80s took America from GPs in solo practice to large managed-care institutions, and forced doctors see a lot more patients more quickly. That produces stress, which in turn gives rise to unprofessional behaviour.

"They're under a lot of stress," says Sylvia Cruess. "They take it out by using a form of humour and funny language which is often derogatory."

In response to factors such as these, organizational heavyweights including the Association of American Medical Colleges and the American Medical Association in the United States as well as the Association of Faculties of Medicine of Canada and the Canadian Medical Association threw their weight behind the principles of professionalism.

The leaders of three powerful groups representing internists from the United States and the European Union started the Medical Professionalism Project, which, in turn, introduced the 2002 Charter on Medical Professionalism. Among its three principles (patient welfare, patient autonomy and social justice) and ten commitments—one of which deals with professional responsibilities—came the admonition to "be respectful of one another."

In the past few years, one medical organization after another has tried to turn the principles of professionalism into policies designed to rid the practice of medicine of unprofessional behaviour. This excerpt from the 2010 Code of Conduct at the University of Illinois at Chicago College of Medicine is typical: "The manner in which we treat each other contributes to effective communication and maintenance of a professional, safe and effective work environment. Our interactions can directly impact patient perceptions of the institution, engagement in their care and willingness to choose us as their preferred care provider.

"Inappropriate communication can create situations where errors are more likely to occur. All individuals have the right to be treated with respect, courtesy and dignity. All practitioners and employees are expected to refrain from disruptive, abusive or otherwise inappropriate behavior towards patients, employees, visitors and other practitioners."

In addition to policies, most medical schools give seminars to incoming students and residents.

"We spend a huge amount of time on inappropriate, unprofessional behaviour," says Richard Cruess. "We talk a lot about the importance of maintaining patient confidentiality and not talking in elevators and hallways in ways that will identify a patient." They also talk a lot about doctors having respect for their patients—and for each other. "Respect is a central tenet of professionalism," he adds.

To the Cruesses, respect means not using slang, or what they call derogatory language. "One of the concerns is the so-called derogatory language that is used, especially during training," says Sylvia Cruess. "Calling a patient a cockroach isn't respectful."

Notice that when it comes to professionalism, the emphasis is on what the doctor says—not what he or she thinks. Sylvia Cruess says the distinction is important.

"What you think is what *you* think, but what you say in public reflects on the whole profession," she says. "So we try and give them a reason for not using this sort of language in public. It may damage the trust that people have in the health-care system and in physicians in particular."

It's unclear to me how thinking something pejorative but not saying it in public is any less damaging than saying it aloud.

In addition to admonishing students and residents, Richard Cruess says there's a new emphasis on rooting out bad role models.

"I'm aware of an institution where a surgeon actually lost his operating privileges because of persistent bad behaviour," he says. "I won't name the institution but the chair of a major department in a major northeast American medical school lost his job because of bad behaviour which didn't appear to be remediable. I'm absolutely positive that would not have happened fifty years ago. Probably not twenty-five, either."

///////

I'm all for rooting out abusive attending doctors. Putting good medical role models into positions of influence seems like a no-brainer as well. But admonishing young ones not to speak disparagingly about patients and each other seems both counterproductive and strangely out of touch.

Do parking tickets get you not to park illegally? How about a tongue-lashing from a parking control officer? Didn't think so. So, then, how do you expect young doctors to respond when the slang police issue them a summons for dishing argot on an elevator? Frankly, anyone who thinks that's going to work doesn't understand the culture of modern medicine.

One woman who does is Dr. Vineet Arora, associate program director for the Internal Medicine Residency at the University of Chicago. Arora is an academic hospitalist who supervises internal medicine residents and medical students, and serves as a career mentor to both. Her research focuses on medical professionalism, resident duty hours, patient handoffs and the quality of medical care. Her blog *FutureDocs* is must reading if you want to understand the culture of medicine that fosters medical slang.

"Professionalism Is a Dirty Word . . . And Why Are Medicine Docs Called Fleas?" That's the headline on a 2010 blog post. Arora wrote that while attending a meeting put on by the Association of American Medical Colleges on how to put quality into teaching hospitals, she heard speaker after speaker asking "how to address the fact that doctors in teaching hospitals don't get along."

Wrote Arora: "Unfortunately, all the specialty bashing that takes place prevents the adoption of a team-based culture necessary to advance quality and safety. As one speaker highlighted, how can we really start to address this topic when specialty services are busy blocking the consult . . . or disparaging the internal medicine doctor by calling them a 'flea'? I hadn't heard the term 'flea' in a while, but many onlookers were nodding in agreement, possibly thinking about the last time they heard someone disparaging the ER for an incomplete workup or a specialist blocking the consult as 'inappropriate.' The discussion about quality and safety morphed into every medical educator's favourite topic, 'professionalism.'"

I can understand that doctors in practice who are long past their medical formative years might reject medical professionalism and embrace medical slang and other forms of patient and colleague disrespect. On the other hand, given the power medical schools wield over students, I'd expect that group to be at the forefront of change. Wrong again, according to Arora.

"Ironically, while medical educators love discussing professionalism, this word has become despised by medical students," she wrote back in 2010. Far from embracing it, Arora says, senior medical students at the school where she teaches regularly lampoon medical professionalism. Arora thinks she knows why. "As you can guess, any efforts to 'teach professionalism' to students seem preachy and insincere."

One man who understands the pushback from students perfectly is Fred Hafferty, director of the program in Professionalism and Ethics at the Mayo Clinic in Rochester, Minnesota. Hafferty is a medical sociologist who, more than anyone, has explored the hidden curriculum of medicine—the stuff that's passed from doctor to doctor yet is seldom, if ever, set down in textbooks.

Hafferty suggested I check out *Absolutely American: Four Years at West Point*, a 2003 book by David Lipsky that follows cadets from raw recruits to graduation. Hafferty says the clear message he got from the book is that breaking the many rules at West Point is what recruits do for fun.

To Hafferty, if medical professionalism is all about the rules, then slang represents breaking them.

"You're not supposed to talk about certain things in elevators," says Hafferty. "I mean, we have signs all over [the Mayo Clinic]. I wouldn't be surprised at all that within environments focused so much on saying the right thing, that saying wrong things in ways that nobody recognizes would be great fun. And I mean that sociologically. If I was a student, it would be great fun to figure out how to dance around this without having faculty realize that they're dancing around."

Duke University respirologist Dr. Peter Kussin has championed the use of slang throughout his career. He worries that professionalism's focus on slang as derogatory ignores its therapeutic value to those on the front lines of medicine. "In the ICU, my greatest fear is that when I crack a joke in front of the [patient] room and everyone laughs—even if the joke has nothing to do with the patient—they're going to assume I'm laughing at their loved one," he told me.

"The inability to laugh on rounds in an environment like our ICU, where there's very little to laugh about, is going be tragic and injurious to safety and to the quality of care. You need to have those moments where you take a little break and reset, and the humour does that and the slang is the quickest way to get to the humour."

More than that, calling in the slang police is like outlawing basements because some get flooded. Telling students and residents to keep slang to themselves may sanitize the public hospital discourse, but it doesn't get at the root causes of slang.

Doctors call obese patients whales because they aren't being taught that obesity is a disease. They aren't given equipment to transport bariatric patients safely. They aren't given the tools to operate on these patients effectively. Instead of banning the slang, why not provide the education and support needed to diagnose and treat bariatric patients?

Instead of condemning slang such as *cockroach* and *frequent flyer*, teach ER physicians and nurses to attack the underlying reasons patients visit ERs over and over and over again. Better still, if the ER isn't the best place to manage superutilizers, then follow my colleague Dr. Jeff Brenner's lead and find one that's better.

If ERs have trouble with geriatric and psychiatric patients, then maybe the solution is to give such patients ERs of their own.

On January 24, 2013, a 32-year-old woman was taken by paramedics to the ER at Gila Regional Medical Center in Silver City, New Mexico. According to a story in the *Silver City Sun-News*, the woman's mother called 911 at 9:30 p.m. and told the dispatcher her daughter was suicidal and had a gun. When the woman was brought to the ER, her clothes were taken off and a female nurse searched the woman, but did not find a weapon. Shortly after, the woman pulled out a gun and shot herself.

Mona Shattell says the Silver City incident is not the only one. In a *Huffington Post* blog entry from February 4, 2013, Shattell, a professor in the School of Nursing at DePaul University in Chicago, wrote that in September 2012, a man shot himself outside an ER in Wichita, Kansas; a month earlier, a man in Stillwater Oklahoma killed himself in an ER restroom.

"Had these individuals instead gone to a *psychiatric* emergency room, or one of a few [in the U.S.] specially designed and staffed, non-clinical settings for persons in emotional crisis, their deaths may have been prevented."

The stakes may not be as high for elderly patients, but a movement to build ERs that specialize in geriatric patients is likewise underway in America.

Better places for undesirable patients, better training and better equipment only go so far. The greater challenge is how to get young doctors to want to treat them. I'm afraid fixing that is a long-term project. Medical schools need to recruit students who love caring for the patients we invent slang to describe. While they're at it, both medical schools and hospitals need to recruit leaders and other role models who enjoy caring for twenty-first-century patients.

If doctors don't take up the call, then the other solution is to find different health professionals who like these patients more than doctors do. In both the U.S. and Canada, young doctors just finishing their residencies are increasingly finding it difficult to secure jobs. The phrase *unemployed doctor*—once considered an oxymoron—has become a reality.

Nurse practitioners (NPs) are registered nurses who have taken additional postgraduate training that enables them to have an enhanced scope of practice that includes diagnosing and treating patients, ordering tests and prescribing medications. NPs are salivating at the chance to pick up the slack.

And while we're at it, I think much of the slang directed by one group of doctors toward another goes back to a fundamental problem: we don't empathize with one another because we don't spend a moment thinking about the challenges other kinds of doctors face. One way to reduce that is to have doctors spend time working in other parts of the hospital.

If I were in charge, I'd retire the slang police. I wouldn't encourage slang, but I certainly wouldn't tell young doctors to keep it to themselves. Instead, I'd listen for it, and especially listen for trends that indicate problems in the local hospital culture that need to be addressed.

I suspect that Vineet Arora already does that. I'm not so sure about other proponents of medical professionalism.

/////////

In writing *The Secret Language of Doctors*, one of the things I set out to do was to figure out the impact women are having on the use of medical slang and the attitudes behind it. It's no secret that more and more women are becoming doctors. A growing number of medical schools have student bodies that are more than half female.

Are female doctors less likely than their male counterparts to use slang? Not based on what residents have told me as I've researched this book. I talked to several male residents who felt that women in medicine are just as likely to invent and use slang as their male counterparts. The women I spoke to seem to agree.

"I think we like to think we're different," says a female resident in OBGYN. "But I don't think we really are. I think we don't use as much sexually based slang, but the slang we use is every bit as dark as what the men use."

The reason is that the conditions that give rise to the use of slang have not changed—especially dealing with patients who are at a very intense time in their lives who have really high needs. The atmosphere is often charged. Not only are young doctors emotionally exhausted, they are physically exhausted as well.

"I think the pressure is huge on women, just as on men," says the female resident in OBGYN. "Sleep deprivation in OBGYN is ridiculous. In the culture, it's almost a competition of how long can you go without sleep. It wears down your soul and your defences."

The only people who really understand that kind of depletion after a night on call are one's colleagues. "The black humour comes in a lot in that case. And I have no doubt it's every bit as much with women as it is with guys."

Richard and Sylvia Cruess think the impact of women doctors on the use of slang can be answered only after a good deal of observation of women in the trenches. Richard Cruess says that, intuitively, women are less likely to use slang.

"I think it depends on the individual," Sylvia Cruess adds. "There certainly are women doctors who are quite derogatory and use derogatory language."

In my opinion, the culture of medicine is strong enough to resist a major gender shift without changing one iota.

///////

On July 15, 2012, Korean singer-songwriter Psy posted "Gangnam Style," a hip-hop song about life among the idle rich who live in a district of the South Korean capital, Seoul. More than 1.7 billion people have watched the video on YouTube—making it the most popular video in YouTube's history. Since then, "Gangnam Style" has inspired hundreds if not thousands of parodies.

One such parody that caught my eye was titled *OB/GYNE Style*, which was written and produced by an OBGYN resident in Toronto.

I liked it immediately for two reasons. First, unlike most of the "Gangnam Style" parodies I've watched, this one was well done. The other reason is that it's filled with OBGYN slang terms like *catching babies*. The resident even says he doesn't mind taking care of morbidly obese women with a BMI of 60.

So proud was Sunnybrook Health Sciences Centre—the hospital where the resident was working at the time the video debuted—that it posted *OB/GYNE Style* to its YouTube channel. The pride and glory were short-lived; Kalina Christoff, founder of Humanize Birth, a group that advocates on behalf of pregnant women, complained in the media that *OB/GYNE Style* was offensive. Soon after, Sunnybrook pulled the video from its YouTube channel.

"People from other obstetrical units were writing in and saying they enjoyed it and that it allowed them to take a light look at their jobs, which can sometimes be a little stressful," Craig Duhamel, Sunnybrook's vice-president of communications, told the *Toronto Star* in a story published on December 23, 2012. "We certainly didn't want to upset anyone—it wasn't our intention at all. While the overwhelming majority of people liked it, there were a few who were upset by it and we wanted to respect their feelings."

In my opinion, the sin of *OB/GYNE Style* was not in producing it, but in sharing it without providing some context.

I, too, have shared lots of medical slang and some inside stories from the people who use slang in everyday hospital discourse. The difference between *OB/GYNE Style* and this book is that I've tried to unpack and explain the culture from which the slang comes. I leave it to you to decide if *The Secret Language of Doctors* should remain in the shadows.

In my view, the major impact of medical professionalism so far is that it has made medical slang more hidden. Before, it was spoken openly in hospital elevators and corridors. Now, it's whispered to trusted friends and colleagues. But it's there and it continues to flourish.

Just ask Dr. Christian Jones, former chief resident in surgery at the University of Kansas Medical Center. Now embarking on a career as a surgeon and helping teach the next generation of surgical MDs, he's proud to say he read *The House of God* and says absolutely he uses slang.

"Some of the medical slang has changed and some of it has not," says Jones. "But it's in use every day, around every patient, on every ward of every hospital. And, while *The House of God* was written in a somewhat different time, there are culture shifts in medicine that are too slow to make anyone think that this has entirely gone away."

///////

More than thirty-five years have passed since *The House of God* was first published. These days, the original slangmeister, Dr. Stephen Bergman, is doing a victory lap—savouring the enduring recognition he and his book have earned.

As I ended my conversation with Bergman at his home in Newton, Massachusetts, I wanted to know what he thought of the fact that thousands—perhaps millions—of physicians know about GOMERs, *turfing, bouncing* and many other slang terms thanks to him. "I like the fact that it helps them," said Bergman. "I really do, because it helped me. I like the [terms] that are helpful in actually getting through the day and GOMER is one of those."

I asked Bergman if it's possible to use slang and still be professional.

"Well, that's the question." Bergman stared out the window of his office on the second floor of the carriage house where he's still turning out novels and plays—grasping for a pithy thought. "I think you just have to get down in the dirt with what's human. It's like when you're meditating. All this crap comes into your mind. You don't say, 'I can't have that crap in my mind,' because that only makes it get bigger. It is just part of being a doctor in that situation."

Suddenly, Bergman's eyes lit up—not the eyes of the intern who in the 1970s pulled back the curtain on hospital culture, but of the psychiatrist who spent much of his career treating patients with alcohol and drug abuse. He had one more bit of wisdom to give me.

"When you're with someone who's secretly an alcoholic or an addict and he or she mentions the alcohol or whatever drug, they'll lick their lips unconsciously," said Bergman. "You give me twenty minutes with somebody and I'll figure out if they're an alcoholic or not."

I asked him if this clinical pearl has a name. He thought about it for a moment.

"I call it the Shem sign," said Bergman, reverting to the pen name he used to write *The House of God*. "I'd love to publish it."

I'm happy to have the honour—an unexpected gift from Bergman, still the slangmeister after all these years.

Acknowledgements

Following the success of *The Night Shift*, I cast about looking for the right book to follow it up. My proposal for a book on medical errors fell somewhat flat, as the marketplace for books on patient safety is quite crowded.

Then, Jim Gifford, my stalwart editor at HarperCollins, made a fateful suggestion. Pointing to the incredible success of the book *How Doctors Think*, by Dr. Jerome Groopman, Gifford suggested I consider writing a book that unpacks how doctors talk. He envisioned a light and breezy volume about the ubiquitous medical jargon that is a staple of television shows such as *Grey's Anatomy* and *Scrubs*.

As I started my research, it soon became clear that I could use the book as an unprecedented lens with which to explore the culture of modern medicine, something I have made a career of on my CBC Radio show *White Coat, Black Art*.

While Gifford thought I would focus on medical jargon, it soon became clear to me that it was medical slang or argot, not jargon, that reveals what doctors think about patients, challenging situations and one another.

To discover contemporary slang, I began my search with the first purveyor of medical slang, Dr. Stephen Bergman (better known by his pen name Samuel Shem), author of the marvellous novel *The House of God*. Bergman filled me in on the origins of the book and the slang to which he introduced readers. As well, his reactions to contemporary slang form a critical part of my book. I am extremely grateful for his generosity and the support he lent the book.

The research for this book would not have got off the ground if not for the support and incredible networking of my friend and colleague Melissa Travis. Melissa, better known in the twitterverse as @ DrSnit, paved the way for me to connect with dozens of health professionals who are also mavens of medical blogs and other avenues of social networking. These include Hood Nurse, Dr. Grumpy and Not Nurse Ratched.

I interviewed dozens of residents of all disciplines, including family medicine, internal medicine, surgery, anesthesia and obstetrics and gynecology. I am grateful to them for their contributions of slang in current use, stories that depict the emotionally charged situations in which the slang is used, and for their candid opinions on difficult patients and difficult colleagues.

I also extend my appreciation to the many attending physicians and other health professionals who gave me their time, their slang, their stories and their passion for the work they do. In particular, I'd like to single out colorectal surgeon Dr. Marcus Burnstein and obstetrician-gynecologist Dr. Raz Moola for their incredible accounts of triumph and tragedy on the front lines.

I am indebted as well to paramedic and stand-up comedian Morgan Jones Phillips, who shared some painful memories of tragedies that occurred at track level in Toronto's subway system.

I also wish to thank Dr. Peter Kussin, a respirologist and critical care specialist at Duke University Hospital, for his stories and for his love of medical argot. I look forward to reading his book on the language of medicine.

There were times during my research that I lost my way and began to doubt the value of my work. Fortunately, at those times, I had a support crew of true believers who helped me see the importance of the book in explaining medical culture. In particular, I would like to acknowledge medical sociologists Renee Fox and Fred Hafferty, whose critical support helped sustain my enthusiasm to complete the book.

The Secret Language of Doctors is a research-intensive project. I could not have found and interviewed by myself the dozens of sources needed to flesh out modern medical argot. I am so grateful that Erin James Abra, a talented young writer and researcher, came on board as my co-investigator of slang, researcher, sometime writer, confidant and friend. Late in the process, Erin's critical comments in response to the first draft of this book made it much better.

I also wish to thank freelance editor Shelley Robertson for fixing the tenses I got wrong repeatedly, and for her enthusiastic comments following each chapter that she edited so lovingly. In the same vein, I'd like to single out Juanita Hadwin for her fast and accurate transcriptions of the many audio interviews that Erin and I assembled in the preparation of this book. Her supportive reactions to the interviews that she transcribed kept me grounded and helped me keep my readership in mind. I am grateful to fellow author and journalist Ann Rauhala for introducing me to both Erin and Shelley.

I'm thankful to my bosses at CBC, Linda Groen, Chris Straw and Chris Boyce, for giving me a national platform on CBC Radio One to explore the culture of modern medicine. I'm also thankful to my colleagues Dawna Dingwall, Jean Kim, Kent Hoffman and Jeff Goodes, whose contributions to *White Coat, Black Art* enriched my understanding of the inner workings of health care.

I wish to express my gratitude to my agent Rick Broadhead, who has given me sound business advice and emotional support well before *The Night Shift* and up until and including *The Secret Language of Doctors*. His warnings on the sophomore jinx were well taken, at least looking back.

I want to thank my editor, Jim Gifford, whose level-headedness and ability to bring out the best in authors is as astonishing to me as is his ability to read and grasp a book in a matter of hours.

About the Author

Brian Goldman is an emergency physician at Toronto's Mount Sinai Hospital and the host of CBC Radio's award-winning program *White Coat, Black Art*. His inspiring yet bracingly honest TEDx talk about medical errors—which has been viewed on the Internet almost 1 million times—has cemented his reputation as one of his generation's keenest observers of the culture of modern medicine. The author of the acclaimed book *The Night Shift*, Dr. Goldman lives in Toronto with his wife and two children.

224
Clinics
Bremner